THE TACTICS OF

Supportive Therapy

A COMPREHENSIVE

INTERVENTION PROGRAM

FOR EFFECTIVE CARING OF

THE ALZHEIMER'S VICTIM

BY LEN FABIANO

SECOND EDITION

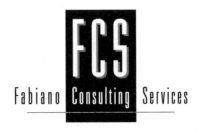

FCS provides a wide range of services to the health care industry including;
in-house seminars, publications and audio-visual material.

For further information and a free catalogue, contact:

Mr. Len Fabiano
FCS President
(705) 786-1747 Canada /(800) 387-8134 US

DEDICATED TO:

My Father, Joe – who taught me the uses of common sense

My Mother, Mary – who instilled in me the needed sensitivity

My Father–In–Law, Harold – who demonstrated to me the
importance of patience

My Mother–In–Law, Bea – who showed me the success of
perseverance

As always to my wife, Linda, my son,
Daniel and my daughter, Kimberly, whose
love and support provides the foundation
for any of my accomplishments.

Acknowledgments,

It is through the struggles of so many of the mentally impaired elderly I have known that I learned of their experience; through the pain of so many families in their attempts to cope, that I learned of the need; and through the hopes and energies of so many professionals that I learned what to do. To all of you my appreciation.

Again I cannot forget Ron Martyn. It doesn't seem to matter what I do or where I am going, Ron is always there. His ability to enhance what I have to offer and to clarify those things that are always cloudy has always impressed me. Thanks Ron.

Len

ABOUT THE AUTHOR

MR. LEN FABIANO started as an orderly and maintenance assistant in a long term care facility. He is now a Registered Nurse with a degree in Psychology from Brock University. Mr. Fabiano has studied at the University of Michigan, and received his Professional Studies in Aging Certificate offered through the Institute of Gerontology. He is a skilled counselor with advanced training in Transactional Analysis. Along with his experience in psychiatric and intensive care nursing, he was the Director of Nursing for a 350 bed Home for the Aged and Project Advisor to the Canadian Council on Hospital Accreditation with Long Term Care. He is an experienced educator who has taught the diploma nursing and health care aide programs at Durham College. While at the college, he was Program Coordinator and lecturer for the three year Gerontological Certificate Program offered through the Continuing Education Department.

Presently, he is President of ECS, Education and Consulting Service and is a renowned Educational Consultant to LTC facilities throughout the country. He has a private practice counselling seniors and their families and is a contributor to the O.A.H.A. manual Does It Really Matter If Its Tuesday?, A Guide to Care for the Mentally Impaired Elderly. Three other texts written by Len Fabiano and available through ECS are:

1. **Working With The Frail Elderly:** Beyond the Physical Disability (second edition)

2. **The Nurse Manager (& Others Too) in Long Term Care**

3. **Mother I'm Doing The Best I Can**, Families of Aging Parents During Times of Loss and Crisis

Contents

What Does It All Mean?

I recently encountered an individual that epitomized for me the essence of this text. While assessing a long term care facility, staff asked if they could introduce me to one of their residents. I was more than pleased to comply. They took me into the room of a 21 year old woman named Dora, who was suffering from hydrocephalus – a state where the pressure created by blockage of cerebral spinal fluid in the brain enlarges the skull. I have encountered individuals like this before, but no one compared to the person I saw in front of me. This young woman was in a single bed. Her head was virtually the width of the bed. Her body was the size of a two year old. What amazed me was that a person so severely disabled could be alive for 21 years.

When I assessed this lady, I could only initiate pupil reaction by shining a light in her eyes. There was no other response, even to pain stimuli. She was severely incapacitated both mentally and physically. What impressed me was that her skin was in perfect condition, there were no reddened areas or ulcerations. Her bed linen was pink and frilly. The wallpaper that covered the walls of her room was feminine and appropriate for a woman of that age. There were rock star posters on the walls. The radio was on with soothing music and the lighting was set at a comfortable level.

For the rest of the day, whenever two staff walked into Dora's room to perform her care, I followed. On each occasion, the staff who approached her, immediately stroked her head and began a conversation. It was obvious that this action on their part was not performed for my sake. It was too natural and spontaneous to be something that was not done on a regular basis.

Even though the staff knew I was a nurse, they did not expose Dora. They drew the sheets back enough to massage her back and head first on the side of the body that they were about to turn her on. They spoke to her the entire time, telling her what they were about to do. There wasn't a reddened area anywhere to be seen on her body. When the staff finished their duties, they brought the bed sheets up just right, set the music and lighting to its normal level and walked out of the room, telling Dora they would be back later.

Once in the hall, I stopped the staff. I asked them "Why did you spend the time with that resident and perform the care in that manner?" They looked at me bewildered and said "I don't understand!" I replied "All you had to do was go into that resident's room, turn her over, rub her back and get out. Why did you do what you did?" Again they looked at me as though I were peculiar and answered "Dora has been with us all of her life. She will be with us until she dies. Our job is to make her as comfortable as possible." What they really said was that they were responsible to provide this resident with the highest level of quality of life possible. How do you teach that? That is compassion, dogged determination, resourcefulness of spirit . . . to its full extent.

Those who demonstrate such character and perception are impressive in the performance of their care, whether they are professional care givers or family members. It is people like these who have assisted me in the development of the second edition of Supportive Therapy. Through their challenges and questions they have encouraged me to hone and further detail a concept that has gained widespread recognition in enhancing the quality of life for the mentally impaired elderly.

You will find the main changes in this second edition is an expansion of all areas, in order to provide a deeper understanding of the complexities of the mentally impaired. Reading this edition will furnish you with more skills that are necessary to define and implement the level of quality of life witnessed with that 21 year old woman.

Supportive Therapy is a blueprint for understanding and caring for the mentally impaired elderly. The tactics described will provide a comprehensive set of strategies needed to effectively care for the Alzheimer victim. As you begin to use the Supportive Therapy approach to care, and experience new successes, do not stop experimenting, there is always more that can be done. As you will be continually reminded, there are no constants or absolutes with the mentally impaired elderly. What works doesn't (always or sometimes). What doesn't work does (sometimes). Supportive Therapy provides you with a breadth of approaches and techniques that can be modified to suit the person and the circumstances. This approach does not make care of the mentally impaired easy. However, it does make some sense of how to accomplish it effectively.

Chapter One

The Starting Point

In all of my texts, I have employed a highly successful writing technique called Guided Imagery. This approach allows the reader to personalize the experience discussed. There is no greater challenge than to employ this technique with this text. There can be no better way to understand the needs of the mentally impaired elderly than to imagine what it would be like to experience the world as they may. This style requires from you a commitment to be involved. To participate in what you are about to read. Do not take the following technique lightly. It is not a mere form of entertainment, but a valuable and powerful tool that will clarify what you read and increase your comprehension of the concepts presented.

The instructions for the process of Guided Imagery are as follows:

Your task is to read the following scenario, adding a slight twist as you read. You will notice certain phrases are broken with a slash(/). The purpose of each slash is to have you pause; internalize what you have just read; form a mental image of what was described; and then move to the next statement. Take your time and work slowly. In this exercise it is important to hear yourself as you read, so that you can see the sequence of events, and feel the consequences as they apply to you. **Hear it, See it and Feel it**.

I want you to imagine the following:

I approach you
Place a blindfold over your eyes
Plug your ears so you cannot hear/
I take you to an unknown destination

Telling you nothing of where you are going or why/

I remove your blindfold and ear plugs
You find yourself in an unfamiliar building/
In a large crowded room with people you have never seen
        before/
I leave with instructions to those in the room not to let you
        leave/

You can find nothing in the room to help you identify your
        location/
The people who confront you speak a language you have
        never heard before/
You find yourself unable to decipher any meaning from
        their attempts to communicate with you/

People are constantly moving about
Some are touching your clothing
Placing you here, then there/
Even when you refuse to follow, they take you/
Your attempts to leave the building are always thwarted
At times their behaviour seems quite bizarre and
        threatening/

It is getting dark
You believe your family should be missing you by now
        and coming to get you
Instead you are taken to a bedroom with two beds in it/
A person lies motionless in the bed by the door
No sound, no reaction to the activities around/
You are stripped of your clothing
And motioned to lie down on the empty bed/
The lights are turned out/

You cannot rest
You hear unfamiliar noises from outside the door/
Periodically in the darkness a figure walks into the room
        with a flashlight
It is shone in your direction
Then the person leaves/

The sun rises/
Someone comes to you
Hands you a bowl with water and two pieces of cloth/
You do not understand what is asked/
The individual takes the cloth, places it in the water
And then moves the cloth to your face
You attempt to stop her but are unsuccessful/

You never know where you are/
Who the people are around you
Faces and things never remain constant/
The fear you experience never leaves you/
Each day the experience is the same/

There can be no more crippling disorder than to be mentally impaired – a loss of the ability to understand the world around you. A time where, no matter what you do or what is done for you, it does not change the chaos you experience. A world where you hope that people do not ask you to understand, but instead understand you.

REMEMBERING THE PERSON

A well–known author and expert in the field of aging criticized a newly published book on the care of the mentally impaired elderly. Her comments basically stated that she felt the text was too strong on the human side of the experience and too weak on the theory and research end. I look forward to her comments about this text.

I do not dispute that research and theory are important. We would not be where we are today without it. However there is a time when we must go beyond the therapeutic level to a much more complex, much more speculative perspective – the individual's world and what he may need to survive in it. We have spent much of our time these past few years attempting to place a therapeutic label on the direction of our care with the mentally impaired elderly. We have taken things that are normal to life and suddenly re–categorized them to fit the therapeutic model we seem to strive for – therapeutic parks, music therapy, pet therapy, touch therapy, intergenerational programs, reminiscent therapy, and on and on.

Our responsibility to the mentally impaired elderly is more complex than any therapeutic model – we are asked to provide for a variety of mentally impaired residents, the highest degree of **Quality of Life** possible. The success of this venture can only be achieved by providing the resident with every opportunity to function at his maximum level, given the weaknesses and the strengths of the individual at any specific time.

This book is written for the caregivers; those who constantly work with the mentally impaired elderly in institutional settings; those who are required to deal with the human side of our residents' lives. Its emphasis is on the day–to–day care that is the major part of our task. This job at times is repetitive. Doing the same task again and again – reinforcing, re–answering, repeating and constantly supporting. The rewards for this diligence are not obvious to those unfamiliar with the complexities of our role.

The goal of this book is to provide you, the caregiver, with an opportunity to place yourself more deeply into the world of your mentally impaired resident; to personalize what that individual may be experiencing and what he may need. The approach identified in this text is a simple one, one that involves an important, often overlooked skill – **common sense**. To satisfy those who must have a label we will call this **Supportive Therapy**. It can be defined as follows – effective caring for the mentally impaired elderly requires identifying the individual's strengths and maintaining them, identifying his limitations and compensating for them. In dealing with both the strengths and limitations of the mentally impaired person, the expectation must always be made that these qualities will change over time, through the course of the disease and under specific circumstances. The fundamental challenge is that this approach must be maintained for the rest of the person's life.

What we are about to undertake is strongly linked to one of the most successful tools we have in dealing with any of our clients – empathy. Empathy allows us to place ourselves behind the eyes of the individual under our care and adjust our approach and interventions accordingly. The more specific we can be in identifying the world of that person in crisis, whether it be an emotional or physical one, the more appropriate our care. This approach becomes crucial with the mentally impaired as well. Empathy gives us the ability to understand what a mentally impaired resident is experiencing, allowing us to adjust our

4

approach and interventions accordingly. Such a perception ensures satisfying our mandate of achieving the ultimate in quality of life for those under our care.

NOTHING WORKS, EVERYTHING WORKS

The difficulty with the mentally impaired resident is simple – there is little commonalty in what each is experiencing. One resident may not be able to remember faces, but can find his room; another cannot find his room, but can remember faces; and a third cannot remember faces nor the location of his room. Much of what we do with the mentally impaired depends on the individual resident. Expecting to know in advance what is required or how to approach that resident leads the caregiver to a high risk for failure.

Reality orientation is an example of how problems can be created. In the past, staff were instructed on what was considered a specific and universal approach of what to say when a resident was confused – correct him. It didn't work. The resident, only minutes later, asked the same question or became aggressive when contradicted. The expectation that this one approach could be universally effective with all residents created considerable frustration in long term care. This attempt to outline in one broad sweep how to deal with a person with organic brain disease did not work. It often sterilized our approach and limited our effectiveness in meeting the needs of the individual resident.

One thing has become clear these past few years in working with the mentally impaired in long term care – there is no formula, there is no one answer on how to deal with the complex problems presented. It has become hard to accept that not everything we encounter in dealing with our mentally impaired elderly can be dissected adequately in any theory; nor can any research give us the specific direction or a universal answer of what to do with a resident and his problems at any given time.

To the "experts" who profess the need to refer to theory and research, I say in our field of long term care there are no "experts". I invite any "expert" to work at the grass roots level for an extended period of time. To work with the same mentally impaired resident for 5 days a week, for 4 years or longer. To work with not just one resident, but 10 in a specific day. Asking each to perform tasks that can be highly threatening – bathing, dressing, activities, meals, etc. In addition to that role, to be required to perform an array of other tasks in that same 8 hour period – housekeeping chores, activity programs, charting and so on. I guarantee that the "expert" would soon experience the same frustrations of most staff in long term care and find it difficult to constantly emphasize the theory and research and downplay the human approach in care.

It is you the caregiver who has the main responsibility to maintain the dignity of the remaining life of an individual who is mentally impaired. It is the awareness of knowing, no matter what your job involves with this resident, nothing works and everything works. You are constantly challenged to analyze what is happening and why, and what to do with it. Without clear–cut textbook directions of what to do, each staff member must be their own expert – placing him/herself in the world of that resident in order to determine effectively what is the best approach or environment given the circumstances of the moment. This need to be flexible in order to adjust to the changes and vulnerability of the person under our care requires a special talent of the responsible caregiver. Ours is a one–sided relationship to be sure – we can expect little direct information from "those in the know" on how to deal with this person at a specific time. Our wins, no matter how small in the eyes of others, are our wins based on our skill and resourcefulness at that time.

KNOWING OUR LIMITS

If we are about to go into the world of the mentally impaired and experience what they experience there is no option but to speculate; to make a professional hunch on what that person may be encountering. Some will say that this book pushes certain inferences to their limit. They will be right. What we are attempting to do is make sense of a world that can only be known to those experiencing the disability and who, unfortunately, are unable to express to us what they see, hear and feel.

Even though the research and theory is limited in its depth and certainty of what is happening to those experiencing the varieties of dementia, it is time to take the theory and make it functional. What is attempted here is to make the world of the mentally impaired take on some rational form to allow us to relate to the disability. The problem is that what the mentally impaired are encountering is often not rational and is beyond anything we can relate to in our normal life.

It is important to establish our limitations. What you are about to read is not necessarily what the mentally impaired are encountering, but how we can make sense of their world in our terms. Issues and concepts will be identified individually and this dissection of the experience will make some of the concepts seem as though they are universal. They are not. What is being described is an overview of what the entire experience of mental impairment can mean. Each individual goes through a specific set of symptoms and behaviours related to the degree and location of the brain damage encountered.

In the following pages and chapters you will experience three important components. The first is the personalized approach of the writings. You are required to participate in this text, to personalize the experience of mental impairment. The scenarios, questions and imagery are important components in the success of this material. Our approach to mental impairment can be no different than our approach to physical disability or emotional assault – we must understand clearly what the individual is experiencing to be effective in our care. Secondly, you will find in these pages all concepts related to the mentally impaired highlighted as they are identified. It is important that these stand out, for they are the basis for all interventions presented. Thirdly, assessment is the most significant aspect in caring for the mentally impaired elderly. Assessment for the caregiver must be functional – it must focus on issues that provide information to direct care. As a result, these assessment tools must relate to what the resident is encountering. Each area of assessment will be presented in relation to the symptoms or behaviours being discussed as well as a chapter on specific assessment mechanisms that can be employed.

This is a caregiver's sense of what is happening and what can be done. There are a number of other texts that can provide you with considerably more information on the biological and technical issues of mental impairment. The purpose of this book is to clearly define our role in providing quality of life to those mentally impaired residents under our care. Take what we began in the first few pages and move closer to the world of the mentally impaired elderly.

THE WORLD OF THE MENTALLY IMPAIRED

GAINING THE PERSPECTIVE

In attempting to personalize what it is like to be physically disabled, there is a popular simulation entitled "Walk–A–Day–In–My–Shoes". In this simulation participants are given a mock disability. Some will have an arm tied to their body to simulate a stroke; others will have their fingers taped together to simulate arthritis and still others their eyes covered to simulate blindness. Such a simulation technique is a very effective exercise to demonstrate what it would be like if one were actually physically disabled.

Those who have experienced such a simulation usually report a dramatic effect – they move from thinking what it is like to actually feeling what it may mean to be disabled for the rest of one's life. A very effective approach for caregivers in gaining further insight into why a resident may withdraw or become aggressive under such circumstances.

How do you simulate mental impairment? There is available no exercise that is as effective as the "Walk–A–Day–In–My–Shoes" simulation. Understanding how a mentally impaired resident may view his world is no easy task. The best that can be done is to compare this experience to something that may be common to many of us.

BEING LOST

Imagine:

> You are walking through the woods sightseeing
> As the afternoon progresses you suddenly realize you are
>   lost/
> You are not sure which direction to go
> You experience a twinge of anxiety and fear/
>
> You keep moving forward
> Hoping to stumble onto something familiar
> You find that the further you go the more lost you become/
> Hours pass, you are getting cold and hungry

> You know if you allowed it, the fear could intensify to an
>   almost panic level/
> As nighttime draws closer there is only one major priority
>   – survival/

A person who is lost will experience five very distinct sensations. The first involves a growing feeling of anxiety and possibly even fear. These feelings require considerable energy to hold under control to prevent them from developing to a panic level. Surrounded by this cloud of anxiety, rational thinking seems restricted as time passes and the fear intensifies. Should that fear turn to panic and take control, one could find oneself walking around in circles, passing the same tree time and time again and not even being aware of it.

In conjunction with this heightened level of anxiety there develops a second experience involving peripheral vision. While sightseeing, you will find your visual field is large and your visual ability quite acute. If during your walk there was a movement off towards your side you would have no difficulty noticing it, stopping to see if it was a deer or something else worth watching. When you are lost your peripheral or side vision wanes. The longer you are lost, the narrower your field of vision becomes. You develop what can be better termed narrowed or tunnel vision – concentrating straight ahead, looking for something that will help you find your way out. I guarantee that after being lost for two or three hours, you could walk around a bend in the trail and come upon a beautiful field of flowers and not even see it. Your attention would be totally focused on identifying where you are going and how to get out of your situation.

Thirdly, you will find a constant urge or need to walk, always moving 10 steps more. The reason for this action is to find something familiar – a stream, a trail, a rock – something that will help you find your way out. You know once you find something familiar, you will be more in control of the situation and as a result your anxiety level will drop dramatically.

The next common experience of most who are lost is to develop an egocentric–type behaviour. If you and I were friends and lost together for a number of hours, how would you respond if I said to you – "I'm cold, I'm scared and I'm hungry"? Would you care? Probably not! It is hard to worry about someone else's problems when you are experiencing the same yourself. This egocentric attitude seems to result in our developing a very small internal world, one that at times involves our taking care of our own feelings and needs over the needs of others.

Lastly, there is a key word that is experienced by those who are lost – survival, am I going to make it through this?

In review then, the components of being lost are

       1. Anxiety almost to panic
       2. Narrowing or tunnel vision
       3. Looking for something familiar
       4. Egocentricity
       5. Survival

That must be exactly what you would experience if you were mentally impaired.

Being mentally impaired is like being lost – living in a world that makes little sense. In such a state, it would seem to you that no matter what you did or where you went, you could not clearly make sense of what is around you. This can be demonstrated easily enough with your own residents. Take a mentally impaired resident who has lived for some time on a specific unit and gained a degree of familiarity. He may not know exactly where he is, but he can find his room and remember certain faces. Place that same resident on a bus for an outing. The chances are good that while on that bus and during the outing his confusion will increase.

To understand the effect, return to that opening scenario in the beginning pages of the book. In that scenario, you were taken to a location and given no reason why you were there. In that setting, you could not understand the people around you. What effect would such an experience have on you the first 24 hours? Your anxiety level would probably be intensified dramatically and we would find you huddled in the corner of a room, misinterpreting everything that was happening to you. How would you be by the seventh day, having to eat, sleep, dress and bathe with people around you who you do not know? Your fear level would increase substantially. By the way, that opening scenario aptly describes the experience of a mentally impaired individual being admitted to a long term care facility.

Family of a mentally impaired resident will attest to this change in behaviour when that mentally impaired individual is moved from the familiar to the unfamiliar. Moving their loved one from home to a hospital or long term care setting often results in a dramatic increase in that person's confusion and a decrease in his ability to function at tasks that were easily completed at home. Once a degree of familiarity is established within the new setting, the person often returns back to being able to perform those tasks once again. This is similar to the experience of being lost in the bush – as anxiety increased your ability to think clearly and analyze information appropriately was impaired. To the mentally impaired, as anxiety increases, mental functioning decreases.

*MOVING FROM THE FAMILIAR TO THE UNFAMILIAR
INCREASES ANXIETY*

AS ANXIETY INCREASES MENTAL FUNCTIONING DECREASES

Many of the mentally impaired seem to always be looking for something familiar – house, spouse, clothing, etc. To look for something familiar in a world that does not make sense is an attempt by the mentally impaired to make some sense of the world around them. If familiarity is found it provides some control, which will in turn provide some sense of security. You can imagine the effect on your anxiety level if when you were lost in the bush for 2 hours, you suddenly came across a candy wrapper that you know you dropped before you became lost.

LOOKING FOR SOMETHING FAMILIAR

The third aspect that makes mental impairment similar to being lost is what occurs to one's peripheral vision. The mentally impaired similarly experience a state of tunnel or narrowed vision. Imagine you are a physically disabled, cognitively well resident and I am mentally impaired walking past you in the opposite direction. You begin to fall forward. Would I stop to help you? The chances are good that I would not. I probably wouldn't even see you. My attention would be concentrated straight ahead, trying to determine where I am and what is going on. The limited peripheral vision of the mentally impaired can be verified in another way as well.

Sit two mentally impaired residents side–by–side and watch what happens? Neither seems to see the other. For the mentally impaired it is difficult to be aware of what is to one's side when required to concentrate continually on what is in front; who just walked into the room; who is shouting; what created that noise; and so on. For many of those who are mentally impaired, side vision is almost non–existent.

The fourth issue involves egocentric–like behaviour – not being able to respond to the needs or feelings of those around. In counselling spouses of mentally impaired older people, I have so frequently heard the comments "My husband and I have been married for over 40 years. During that time if I was ever sick, he would be there to help me. If I was hurting emotionally, he would always hold me. Ever since he became impaired, it doesn't matter how sick I am he doesn't help. It doesn't matter how much I am hurting, he never holds me." He can't. It becomes almost impossible to be aware of what someone else is experiencing when you cannot deal with what you are going through yourself. As a result, the mentally impaired seem to be drawn into their own world and are oblivious to the feelings of others.

EGOCENTRIC BEHAVIOUR

Lastly is the element of survival. The main priority in such a circumstance is in determining how to exist in a world you cannot understand. You must use whatever limited cues and information makes sense to you to give some degree of control over what you are experiencing. You will attempt to make sense of that world to the best of your ability in order to survive.

SURVIVAL BECOMES THE KEY

Return to the scenario of being lost in the bush.

Shortly after you become lost
I appear/
You have never seen me before/
During the entire time you are lost

I stay 40 steps behind you/
You walk forward
I follow you/
You walk towards me
I go the other way/
When you try to speak to me
I do not answer/
How would this situation make you feel?

Your anxiety level would dramatically intensify. Your mind would race trying to figure out who I was and what I wanted. Now your energies are not only concentrated on finding your way out, but trying to analyze my actions as well. It is amazing how poorly we can analyze an unknown stimulus when our fear or anxiety level is high.

Return to the simulation of being mentally impaired and a resident in a long term care facility. As a staff member, I have been in your room performing care from 0730 hours until 0800 hours. At that time I left and returned again at 0845 hours to take you to the bathroom. Would you remember me? Given that you experience memory loss and cannot remember faces, probably not! I walk to your side; standing next to you I look down at you asking "Do you have to go to the bathroom?" Without any other direct contact or other cuing, would you know who I am talking to or what I am saying? Highly unlikely! This scenario demonstrates another basic concept involving the mentally impaired – if the stimulus is not intense enough it will be missed or misinterpreted.

IF THE STIMULUS IS NOT INTENSE ENOUGH,
IT WILL BE MISSED OR MISINTERPRETED

When I asked if you had to go to the bathroom in the manner described above, you probably would not answer. I then take you by the arm and attempt to stand you up. You respond to my actions by resisting and becoming aggressive. Without the appropriate warning, you do not know who I am or what I want. To you, I am a stranger, pulling you from your chair. You feel out of control, causing your anxiety to intensify to a panic level.

There is little difference between this encounter and the earlier scenario where I followed you through the bush while you were lost. In both circumstances an unknown stimulus was presented at a time when you already experienced considerable anxiety. Your only logical response under such circumstances would result in your becoming defensive, becoming aggressive either physically or verbally in order to protect yourself.

BEING ON DEMEROL

Many of us have been a patient in a hospital sometime through our life and some have required an analgesic (pain killer) like demerol or morphine during that stay. On any of these narcotic drugs an individual loses the ability to retain and analyze information. Some have even reported being unable to remember those hours or days when they were on such a drug.

Imagine:

You are a patient in hospital
You are given 100 milligrams of demerol
Every 3 or 4 hours
For three days/
During that time nothing is clear to you/
Your ability to think is dramatically impaired/
While under the influence of Demerol
I approach you in your hospital room
And ask you to find your car in the hospital parking lot/

Just a minute/
I will even provide you with a floor plan of the hospital/
Spend 45 minutes mapping out your path from your room
Through the hospital corridors
To the front lobby
To the exact spot where your car is/
Now go/

No matter what preparation you are given, there is no possible way to remember what you were told to allow you to find your way through such a maze. Given the medication dispensed, your mental functioning ability would be limited. You would have difficulty analyzing the information provided and retaining what was said.

14

Is there any difference in the experience of a mentally impaired resident attempting to move around a large unit to find his room? He is being asked to function at a very complicated and abstract level when cognitive ability is severely limited. Such restrictions in problem solving ability limit a resident's ability to effectively think and resolve the many different situations encountered. This person is no longer normal in an environment that is not normal.

NO LONGER NORMAL IN AN ENVIRONMENT THAT IS NOT NORMAL

UNDERSTANDING THE PRESSURES

Most of us can relate better to things we can see, than those we cannot. If you have ever worked on a psychiatric unit or had contact with patients with a mental disorder you can attest to this. In dealing with a schizophrenic, manic–depressive, or a chronically depressed patient, it is always a challenge in deciding – is the behaviour we are seeing now part of the disease or a subjective behaviour that the patient can control?

Most of us find it easier to relate to a visible limitation like a physical disability – such as stroke, arthritis, Parkinson's, etc.

Imagine:

I had a stroke/
Experiencing total right sided paralysis
Totally incapable of moving my right arm and leg/
Would you ask me to feed myself with my right hand?

You wouldn't! The obvious response would be to feed me or to teach me to use my left hand.

If I am mentally impaired and disoriented to place
or time due to brain damage, why do you ask me
what day is it today, or where do you live now?

Return to my being physically disabled :

I have a right sided stroke,
A dead right arm/

What would be the effect of repeatedly saying to me –
"Len, pick up your fork with your right hand!
Pick up your fork with your right hand!"/

My frustration and subsequent anxiety would increase dramatically. If I had the tendency to withdraw from such pressure, I would. If I had the tendency to be aggressive – watch out! In fact anyone making such a request would be challenged immediately on the inappropriateness and told the approach was wrong and harmful.

Return again to my being mentally impaired – unable to remember place or time due to brain damage. What would be the effect of repeatedly asking me – "What day is it today? Where are you now? What day is it today? Where are you now?"

The frustration of being asked to perform at a level that is beyond my functional ability would result in increasing my anxiety to a panic state. If I had a tendency to withdraw from such pressure, I would. If I was more apt to be aggressive – watch out! More importantly, few would see the inappropriateness of such an approach and challenge those who make it.

It is important when discussing the mentally impaired to emphasize to all in contact with this person – this is brain damage and what is lost is lost. Once an ability his been eliminated by the destructive process of the diseases, it cannot be relearned. Pressuring this person to function at a higher level will only result in an inappropriate behavioural response.

Given the permanency of the damage that can occur, there can be only one mandate in care – identify the individual's strengths and maintain them; identify his limitations and compensate for them. The foundation of Supportive Therapy.

Such an approach does not attempt to draw or pull from the mentally impaired information, but constantly provides the information needed. A resident who cannot remember where he is needs staff to constantly reinforce that with him. For the resident who cannot remember faces, it is essential that all staff introduce themselves to this resident on every contact, as though every contact was the first (as it is to this resident).

That sounds so simple and basic, but it is not. The difficult issue for the caregiver is that we are required to perform that task for that resident for the rest of his life. The repetitiveness in caring for the mentally impaired is one of the most frustrating aspects of our role. It is one thing to say in theory what is to be done, it is another thing when applied in practice. Working with a resident on a day–by–day basis for months or even years and constantly repeating and repeating is frustrating. It is easy to lose the perspective of this resident. Working with a person so intensely, for so long, being in constant contact sets an expectation that the resident should have the same familiarity with you and what you do, as you have with him and how you do it. There is no guarantee of such familiarity with the mentally impaired elderly in an environment of intense stimulation and change.

LOOKING TO THE PAST

In the sixties and earlier, whenever we discovered an older person showing signs of confusion and disorientation, the descriptive term commonly used was "Senility". In the early seventies there was a reluctance to use that term; such older people were then referred to as having "Senile Dementia". That soon became a label. Every older person showing any degree of mental impairment was soon toting that term on their diagnostic record.

In the late seventies we adopted a new set of words "Organic Brain Syndrome: Acute & Chronic" (interesting that whenever this diagnosis was used, I never saw the term "acute", only "chronic"). Soon it too was destined to take on the same path as the previous two, being applied to any old person showing any degree of cognitive dysfunction. It usually resulted in there being an absence of significant testing and aggressive assessment due to the irreversible nature often associated with such a diagnosis.

Now we have the words "Alzheimer's Disease". A question I ask of many staff of long term care facilities is – "Do you have any older person showing signs of mental impairment that does not have the diagnosis of Alzheimer's?" The usual reply is "**NO**".

I am not implying that Alzheimer's Disease does not exist. Our problem is that it too has become as much a label as any other of the previously used diagnostic terms of the past. In fact many physicians are reluctant to use the term due to the qualities it possesses. As a result there now seems to be two new ones used in the absence of Alzheimer's. This one I truly like – "Alzheimer's–Like Syndrome". The other is "Dysfunctional Brain Syndrome". Again each of these terms may have a significant and specific meaning in the diagnostic circles, but in the practical world they have been misused and abused.

Set the scenario in the following manner:

> You are driving your car/
> You drive into your driveway, get out of your car
> You can't find your house/
> Even though it is right in front of you,
> You can't recognize it or your street/
> Your family and neighbours come to you,
> You can't recognize any of them/
>
> You are taken to emergency/
> Guaranteed your physician would do every test imaginable
> to determine the problem/
> If your doctor cannot find the cause of your confusion and
> disorientation,
> He and your family or both may demand a specialist
> Another hospital with better and more sophisticated
> equipment/
> Even if that doctor could not find the answer,
> Your family may still demand another hospital
> Another doctor/
>
> I will make you 78 years old
> You are taken to emergency confused and disoriented/
> What happens?

It very much depends on your doctor and the hospital where you are taken. If your doctor's attitude is positive in terms of investigating the cause of your symptoms and the needed resources are readily available, assessment will be thorough and complete. If your doctor believes that what you are experiencing is probably chronic and little can be done due to your age, then aggressive assessment will probably be withheld. A diagnosis of irreversible brain disorder will be applied. You will be medicated and placed on the waiting list for long term care.

This problem results from the simple fact that there are few physicians who really understand the elderly, let alone Alzheimer's disease. The restriction of aggressive assessment due to age is still a common experience for many seniors. Inappropriate and inaccurate ordering of medications, lack of counselling and emotional support for significant losses have lead to a simple alternative when that one symptom "confusion" is encountered – Alzheimer's.

Few of our centres have the equipment or expertise to diagnosis Alzheimer's. If you are living in a large metropolitan area the chances are good that geriatricians and assessment clinics are available. Unfortunately, these are probably saturated, allowing only priority cases in for thorough assessment. More significantly, it is the general practitioner who must refer people to these centres and if his knowledge or attitude towards the elderly is restrictive, so is his treatment. I have a favorite question I ask physicians when I encounter a roadblock in adjusting medication or attempting an assessment due to the physicians belief that all that can be done has been done given the person's age – if this individual were 45 would your stopping in the assessment process be acceptable. If the answer is yes then fine, if no, then why stop because the person is 78?

We will discuss the causes of mental impairment shortly, but it is important to establish that we still have a long way to go to ensure that treatment and assessment of the elderly experiencing mental dysfunction is universal in its approach and resources applied. To prove this point, let us look at the numbers: approximately 60% of those who are mentally impaired experience Alzheimer's Disease, 20% Multiple Infarct Disease and the last 20% Primary Treatable Causes of Confusion & Disorientation (previously called Acute Organic Brain Syndrome). Presently, there are only two ways to diagnose Alzheimer's – a complete work–up including a blood work series, x–ray series, spinal tap, CAT scan, neurological and psychological assessment or an autopsy after death. How many of your residents who are diagnosed Alzheimer's have had this kind of work–up, or even an autopsy at death to confirm the diagnosis?

The numbers may be even more skewed than presently identified. In certain areas where resources may not be available for proper diagnosis or where the treating physician does not believe aggressive action on his part is necessary due to the patient's age, the number of misdiagnosed mentally impaired elderly residents may be even higher.

We still have a long way to go.

Chapter Two

The Disease

INTRODUCTION

There is a tendency by some family members and even professional caregivers to want Alzheimer's packaged into neat answers and predictions so that programming and care can be easily defined. The biological changes, cause, effects, results, course, etc. of this disease provides no such luxury. Research and the understanding of this disease process itself are still at an infancy state. The reality is that there is probably more that is not understood about this type of mental impairment than we understand. This is not a criticism of the researchers, but an emphasis on the challenges presented when caring for an Alzheimer's victim.

It is important to stress that this disease is highly unpredictable. Understanding what is happening to the brain and the person is speculative at best. At present Alzheimer's disease can only be diagnosed by autopsy or by a process of elimination. (ruling out every possible treatable disease by thorough testing). When nothing else can be found that could cause the person's symptomology, then the conclusion is it must be Alzheimer's. That, in itself, demonstrates the uncertainties this disease presents.

What complicates it even further is that we are not dealing with a disease process that is a separate entity of its own. There are many factors that influence mental functioning – emotional state, past intelligence level, effects of other diseases, drugs, sensory loss, etc. Combine any one or more of these factors with the unpredictable pattern of Alzheimer's and you clearly understand the challenges faced in attempting to define what is happening and what may happen.

Do not look here for neat, packaged answers about the disease process. The emphasis of this book is not on a disease, but on effective care strategies. The information presented about this disease is intentionally condensed to ensure that a basic understanding of the biological process is established. This assures that the rationale for the interventions presented in the later chapters are understood. If further information is needed concerning the medical research and theory, then it is important that one looks to other sources.

One factor must continually be stressed – regardless of the cause, biological changes or the course of the disease, our mandate remains constant – to provide to the Alzheimer's victim the greatest level of quality of life for the remaining years available. The philosophy behind Supportive Therapy.

UNDERSTANDING ALZHEIMER'S DISEASE

1) The Biological Changes

When most think of damage to the brain at an older age, they often associate it with a dysfunction in the circulatory system. With Alzheimer's that is not so much the case. This disorder causes a dysfunction in the electrical conduction system of the brain or how nerve cells or neurons within the brain communicate.

What seems to occur is a change in the manner in which messages are transmitted from one brain cell to another due to physical changes occurring in each neuron. The disease causes certain neurons to deteriorate, taking on a peculiar shape and eventually losing their ability to function.

Microscopic views of damaged neurons show nerve cells that "appear to be tied into knots", these configurations are called neurofibril tangles. At some point these cells are completely destroyed causing black patches of dead tissue throughout certain regions of the brain called senile plaques.

These changes can cause varying degrees of destruction and can be located anywhere in the brain. The predominant areas seem to be the temporal and frontal lobes, and the heart of the brain called the hippocampus. This presents an important consequence relevant to caring for an Alzheimer's victim. The location and degree of damage is individualized. This dictates that no two Alzheimer's victims are identical in the degree and location of destruction within the brain. Therefore no two Alzheimer's victims will experience the same intensity and pattern of symptoms. As a result programming needs are also individualized. What will work for one Alzheimer's victim, may not work for another.

THERE ARE NO TWO ALZHEIMER'S VICTIMS THE SAME,
THEREFORE CARE STRATEGIES ARE HIGHLY INDIVIDUALIZED

2) The Cause

At this time, the cause of Alzheimer's is unknown. It depends very much on which researcher you follow when considering the primary cause of this disease. Some have linked the changes in the brain to alterations in the genetic material of each cell resulting in the cell virtually withering and dying from within. Others have associated it with the impact of a slow acting virus. Some have contributed it to a high aluminum content in the brain of Alzheimer's victim's. Still others have linked it with the decrease in production of a neurotransmitter substance called acetylcholine missing or in limited supply in the nerve cells of the brain. Still others . . . The research continues.

3) The Effect

What is most significant about this disease is that it is brain damage to the fullest extent. Nerve cells are destroyed and lost. The destruction can be so intense for some Alzheimer's victims that an autopsy could reveal a 40% decrease in brain size and weight due to the loss of neuronal tissue. This one fact alone emphasizes one of the most significant frameworks in any philosophy dealing with Alzheimer's disease – what is lost is lost, you cannot put it back.

WHAT IS LOST IS LOST

Alzheimer's is a progressive, deteriorating disorder causing mental functioning to drop over time until death (see diagram #1). There is no way to slow this disease, cure it or stop it. In fact in assisting family to understand and cope with the effects and progression of this disease, it is often helpful, even though hard to accept, to compare Alzheimer's disease to terminal cancer or Multiple Sclerosis. This demonstrates the permanency and progressive nature of the disease.

The permanency of the destruction is an important factor in evaluating any care intervention. If you are able to eliminate a symptom of an Alzheimer's victim with something other than medication, then it is probably not Alzheimer's disease that is causing it.

IF YOU ARE ABLE TO ELIMINATE A SYMPTOM OF THE DISEASE WITH SOMETHING OTHER THAN MEDICATION, THEN IT IS PROBABLY NOT ALZHEIMER'S DISEASE THAT IS CAUSING IT.

The reality is that all you can do when caring for an Alzheimer's victim is to learn to live with the effects of the disease and assist the person to function to the best of his ability regardless of the circumstances.

The irreversible and progressive nature of this disease substantiates the basic premise for the philosophy of Supportive Therapy – identify the person's strengths (what is still remaining) and maintain them and his limitations (what is lost) and compensate for them.

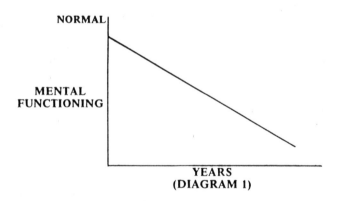

(DIAGRAM 1)

THE COURSE OF ALZHEIMER'S DISEASE

Alzheimer's disease can effect individuals as young as 40. It appears, the younger the individual, the more severe and rapid the deterioration. Like everything else with this disease, there is no certainty, but the pattern seems to suggest that the <u>average</u> life

24

expectancy of a younger person (the period from onset of the disease until death) is about two years.

The age group we more often encounter involves those over 60. The <u>average</u> life expectancy of an individual in this age group with this disease is about 8 years. Some have been known to live as little as two years and others as long as twenty years plus.

It is difficult to pinpoint the exact length of the disease for any individual. The onset of this disease is extremely insidious or slow. Given that the symptoms often develop gradually and initially can be easily hidden, accurately identifying when it began is no easy task.

In fact when discussing Alzheimer's disease, we can divide its course into three levels. These levels should not be confused with the phases or stages of the disease. The stages of the disease describe the biological process that may be occurring. These levels define the person's functioning ability and the resultant care that is needed.

Alzheimer's Disease – <u>Level One</u>

This represents the initial effects experienced by the disease. During this time the individual may not be diagnosed or even suspect that he may be ill. Even though he soon becomes aware that something may be wrong, he is often unwilling to admit that it is anything serious.

In fact, at the beginning or onset of the disease, few who associate with this individual are even aware that there is anything seriously the matter. The symptoms are much too subtle and the progression too insidious to create alarm. It is only when the victim does something very peculiar that the family becomes concerned and seeks medical attention.

Imagine:

      I am 78 years old
      Your father
      Living with you in your home/
      We are sitting in your kitchen
      I am attempting to balance my bank statement/

I find I can't do it
It is not just the bank statement that is the problem
The numbers just don't make sense/
A month ago I had little problem with this task
Now adding simple numbers seems impossible/
Instead of expressing concern
I innocently pass you the book
Stating "I can't seem to get this to balance with my
      cheques,
Would you check it for me?"/

Father seems to always have a reason for his inability – he is over tired, it's too complicated, he just needs help, he is thinking about something else and can't keep his mind on what he is doing . . . an endless list of excuses. In actual fact he is merely camouflaging his difficulties. Afraid or reluctant to admit that his "mind is failing".

Normally there is little alarm on the family's part – a 78 year old father having trouble making the bank statement balance is not unusual. In fact most of us experience that problem from time to time. Family are not quickly conscious of the recurring pattern of father's limitations. They simply attribute it to a slight forgetfulness or unfortunately stereotype his behaviour as simply "old age". In actual fact, father has difficulty with all numbers.

To your spouse he states – "I keep getting the numbers of your address mixed up with my old one at home. What are they again?" Or to one of the kids "What's the last three digits of our phone number, it's slipped my mind again. And the first, and second? That's right!" Sounds more like he is correcting you than not remembering himself.

At this point members of the family are usually not alarmed. They do not collaborate and identify a pattern in dad's inability to function as he used to – only a 78 year old dad who is having some trouble remembering things. It is not until some peculiar behaviour – wandering onto the street and getting undressed – does the family become alarmed and take dad to the doctor.

Once the doctor has completed a thorough examination and ruled out any treatable cause for his impairment, he then makes the diagnosis of Alzheimer's disease. He will explain to the family the progression and characteristics of the disease. It is then that the family pull it all together, often exclaiming "Good Lord, this may have been going on with dad for years but we didn't see it!"

It is not unusual for family members to question "Had I brought dad to the doctor two years ago when it first began, would it have made a difference?" The answer of course is no. There is no treatment for the disease or a way of slowing the progression. Unfortunately some family members may not accept that response. They needlessly feel guilty for not doing something earlier, even though nothing could have been done to change the situation.

A resident of a long term care facility can easily be identified at this functioning level. This is the person frequently found walking the halls. If you ask her "Mary are you having trouble finding your room?" She will often respond "Well . . . no! I know I am going in the right direction, aren't I?" This person is experiencing an increasing difficulty remembering where she has put things or where she is going but can function normally in almost every other sense. Yet she frequently denies that she has any problems.

At level one the person not only experiences an increasing degree of anxiety, but a considerable amount of frustration as well. This frustration arises from the fact that the person knows he could perform a certain task or easily remember things only a short while ago, but as time passes he finds it harder and harder to maintain those abilities.

An Alzheimer's victim at level one requires little physical care, only specific supports to deal with those things that give him the greatest difficulty. In fact it is not the symptoms that create the problems as much as the associated emotions. This person demonstrates frequent and abrupt emotional swings that can create significant problems for family and professional caregivers.

Imagine how you would feel if you discovered or suspected seriously that you had Alzheimer's disease. You would go through every stage of the grieving process:

Denial   – "I am not sick, there is nothing wrong with me."
Blaming   – "Why are people always hiding things on me."
Bargaining   – "Maybe if I eat only certain foods or take
                   vitamins or herbs I can make it better."

Depression   – "I give up there is nothing left for me to do."
Anger   – "This shouldn't be happening to me."
Acceptance   – "I must get on with what remains of my life."

Grieving is experienced as the result of encountering any loss. As the disease progresses and the person's functioning deteriorates further, he experiences further loss in ability. At this level the person is fully aware of what he loses and responds accordingly.

Unfortunately, this disease does not remain static. It is always changing. A person at this level may initially begin forgetting the location of things. He looks for a cup in the kitchen. He starts at the first cupboard where he thinks it is. It's not there. His anxiety is increasing over his inability to find it. He goes to the second cupboard where he believes the cup may be, again it is not there. He becomes frustrated further. He goes to the third cupboard, it is still not there. Now he is very angry and slams the cupboard closed. Unfortunately the cup is in the forth cupboard he opens, but by this time he is so angry with himself that he doesn't see it. He slams the cupboard closed and moves to the next cupboard.

To prevent a person at this level from losing control, things cannot be left to memory. Therefore cue cards are used. These are small cards that are placed on cupboard doors, dressers and closet doors, listing by word and picture what is behind that door. This prevents the need to continually search to find the item. He simply reads the cards.

Unfortunately, many of my clients initially do not call these cue cards. They call them "idiot cards". To ask a 78 year old man to use little cards like a two year old can be degrading, a major assault on one's independence and self image. This simple intervention will initiate any or all of the stages of grieving. Hopefully, after a period of time, he will understand the importance of such a supportive device and finally admit to himself that he can no longer function by memory to find the things he needs and will use the cards. He has reached the stage of acceptance. The very next day he cannot remember his daughter's name, a new loss. The grieving process and emotional swings will begin again.

These emotional swings are the hardest for family and caregivers to deal with. In fact the wife will frequently complain "why is it that my husband always makes a scene, yet he doesn't want anyone to know he has the disease?" In this situation the husband tries in each situation to act "normal", but when he loses control, he loses control of his emotions as well.

Imagine:
> You and I are married/
> I have been diagnosed with the disease
> I do not want anyone else to know/
>
> We have company over for coffee
> Everything is proceeding normally/
> I mention to our guests
> "Did Mary tell you that last October
> the basement flooded . . ."
> I proceed to tell our company an accurate account of the
> details of that incident/
> Not five minutes after I finish
> I interrupt again by stating
> "Did Mary tell you that last October
> the basement flooded . . ."
> Again I recall the story in full/
> The company smiles/
> Only five minutes later, I interrupt the conversation again
> "Did Mary tell you that last October
> the basement flooded . . ."
> Telling the story at length once again/
> The company stares at the ceiling or shakes their head/
> When I notice their response
> I get angry and pound my fist on the table/
> I turn to you and yell
> "I am sick and tired of these people, don't invite them here
> again!"/
> I storm out of the room/

In this situation the husband is not intentionally "making a scene", but responding to his loss of control. At this level he quickly forgets what he has just said, resulting in his frequently repeating himself. Unfortunately his cognitive ability is high enough that he is able to identify by the response of those around that he must have done something wrong even though he does not know what it was. At that point he becomes angry with himself, loses control and lashes out to those around him.

One of my major concerns of a client at this level is the possibility of suicide. When this person is aware that he has the disease and knows what may be in store for him as it worsens, then the future holds tremendous fear. Suicide attempts at this level may not be overt or obvious (hanging or by shooting) but covert or hidden – over-medicating one's self, falling down stairs, car accident, etc. With a car accident it only takes a second too decide "I have had enough" and pull the wheel.

This is not intended to elicit undue alarm by family or caregivers causing them to read every act or incident as an attempt to commit suicide. All aspects and effects of this disease must be discussed, even though they may be very painful or too difficult to admit.

This raises the issue, should a person diagnosed of Alzheimer's disease be told he has it? Return to our earlier scenario when we compared this disease to other terminal illnesses. If a person had terminal cancer, would you tell that individual? If the answer is "no I wouldn't", it is unfortunate. How can you help a person overcome some of the symptoms if the person does not know what is happening? One thing that will be emphasized again and again throughout this text is that an Alzheimer's victim regardless of his functioning level cannot be allowed to lose control. Once control is lost, anxiety increases and mental functioning will be further impaired. Supports are required to compensate for what is lost in order for the person to function at his maximum level. If you don't tell him he has the disease, how do you place the cue cards around the house?

I remember a man in his late forties who sat in one of my presentations on Alzheimer's disease. He and his wife approached me at the end of the session and he told me he had just been diagnosed with the disease. I responded "Whatever you want to say to your family or do to ensure that things are taken care of, you must do it now!" He responded "You are scaring me!" I told him that he could not wait, there is no way to predict what will happen and when. He must resolve issues while he is still able to function, as would any person who knew he would die soon. The realities of this disease demonstrates the harshness of its effects and the difficulties in coping.

In fact a common concern that I have heard from those at this level is "It is not just the disease that scares me, but knowing that at some point during the disease I will no longer be in control of my own dignity, but must rely on others to control it for me." I have just revealed to you a personal commitment that I have made to those at this level of functioning, which is reflected continually in the concepts of Supportive Therapy – a vow to respect that person's dignity regardless of ability.

Alzheimer's Disease – Level Two

An Alzheimer's victim at this functioning level is often physically well, ambulatory, demonstrating considerable wandering and aggressive behaviour and is very confused and disoriented. Mentally this is an individual in frequent conflict. This person seems to be aware of two worlds existing at the same time – theirs and reality as we know it.

Imagine:
I am mentally impaired
Living on your unit/
Being disoriented
I believe that I work here or am only visiting/
At 3 p.m. staff head for the door to go home/
I follow/

When I reach the door
One of the afternoon staff stops me
Stating "Len, you have to stay, this is where you live."/
I respond angrily
"I don't live here. I'm going home."
I fight to push past her./

This person's confusion and disorientation results in his not knowing where he is. He may believe that he is not a resident of a long term care facility, but only a visitor. When he sees staff leave to go home, he follows. Being stopped and told this is his home, causes him to be further confused. His confusion causes a feeling of being out of control, his anxiety level is increased to a panic state, he becomes aggressive or wanders as a result. At level two this person has enough comprehension to know what is being said or is aware of certain aspects of what is happening, but what is said or happening is in conflict with what he believes.

In the upcoming chapters it will be frequently demonstrated that the world of the mentally impaired is real to

31

them. Our challenge is to better understand that person's reality in order to adapt our interventions accordingly. It is those in level two of functioning that pose the greatest challenge to the caregiver.

A person in level two responds differently to surroundings and circumstances than level one. As demonstrated earlier, those in level one are still aware of the subtle cuing available in the environment. Level two does not have that degree of comprehension. As a result, his response to situations are dramatically different.

Imagine:

> You and I are married/
> I have been diagnosed with Alzheimer's disease
> It has now progressed to level two/
>
> You have company over for coffee/
> I sit down and join you
> Immediately I interrupt the conversation stating
> "Last October the basement flooded."
> You respond "Yes dear."/
> Two minutes later, I interrupt the conversation again
> "Last October the basement flooded."
> You respond again "You've just told us that."/
> "Yes, but the basement flooded."
> The company smiles/
> "Last October the basement flooded."
> The company stares at the ceiling and shakes their head/
> "Last October the basement flooded."
> Finally they excuse themselves and leave/

At this level the person is no longer capable of picking up the subtle cuing of facial expressions and body movements from those around to indicate that something is wrong. He has very severe memory loss and cannot remember what he just said as soon as he said it. He goes on repeating himself until he clears the room and even then may still continue.

The only time a person in level two of functioning may become frustrated and possibly be aggressive is if family continually tell him that he is repeating himself or try to stop him, rather than ignoring his behaviour. Family no longer deal with the emotional outburst seen with level one, but now must cope with the repetitiveness and their own possible frustration for not being able to stop it.

This is not to suggest that a person at level two is oblivious to his environment. There are certain aspects of his surroundings that he will respond to and others that he cannot interpret or even perceive. This person is very vulnerable to his surroundings and the events that occur around him. The majority of this text is dedicated to understanding what an individual at this level may be experiencing and the necessary strategies required in his care.

Alzheimer's Disease –Level Three

A person at this level of functioning is incapacitated both physically and cognitively. Physically this person requires complete care – being fed, washed, dressed and is totally immobile. Mentally this person seems oblivious to the world around him. He appears not to be aware of a person's presence until he is touched. Even then he probably does not understand the content of what is said or who is saying it. This person responds mainly to basic stimuli. If yanked roughly out of a chair or talked to in a loud and aggressive voice, he will instinctively jerk back or become afraid. Those in level three require total care and respond to limited programming.

Yet, it is the person in level three who best represents the cornerstone to the basic philosophy in effectively caring for the mentally impaired elderly.

Imagine:
> Your mother is in a car accident/
> She is admitted to an Intensive Care Unit in hospital
> She is totally unconscious and on all life supports/
> As the ICU nurse,
> How would you want me to treat your mother while she
>   was in that state?

The answer is obvious. Staff would be expected to treat your mother as though she could understand what was happening around her.

Only a small percentage of what is in our mind is at the conscious level. A much larger portion is in the unconscious. Even though a person at level three seems oblivious to what is going on around him, we do not know what that individual can see, hear, feel or understand. Given that fact, it is mandatory that we treat this person with the expectation that everything and anything can be understood, even though the person cannot indicate that is the case. The expectation of anyone in contact with an Alzheimer's victim is to treat that person as a normal functioning adult, but not to expect normal behaviour.

It will be emphasized repeatedly in the following chapters that the way this person is perceived and treated will play a substantial part in how this person acts. If an Alzheimer's victim is treated as a child, he will probably respond with child-like behaviour. If he is treated as though he were "crazy", he will probably present "crazy-like" behaviour.

There is nothing more irritating than to watch two staff or two family members standing over an Alzheimer's victim, talking about him. It is no wonder the person is agitated. Appropriate programming (what is required to ensure effective care) at this level can be compared to the concept of palliative care.

It is well known that when a person is dying and unconscious, it is extremely valuable for family or a caregiver to sit with that individual, stroking his hand and talking to him. Physical and emotional security must be provided regardless of a person's functioning level. When dealing with level three, it can only be communicated by the most basic of means.

From a functioning standpoint these three levels can be summarized in the following manner:

Level One
- in contact with reality
- few lapses in mental functioning
- able to respond to programming and activities of daily living well with minimal supports
- experiencing significant emotional swings
- undergoing intense grieving.

Level Two
- ambulatory
- generally physically well

34

- main care challenges are behavioural, wandering and/or aggressive outbursts
- in contact with two distinct worlds, theirs and reality as we know it
- has difficulty performing activities of daily living
- all programming must be adapted to meet his specific level of mental functioning
- significant supports are required
- the environment must be controlled to decrease the amount of stress and stimuli encountered.

Level Three
- exists mainly in whatever world is retained in his mind
- generally oblivious to what is outside him except for very basic stimulus like touch, sound, voice tone, etc.
- requires total care in activities of daily living
- does not respond well to programming that requires cognitive functioning.

[Note: Generally Alzheimer's disease, is at this point, not considered the cause of death. The disease causes such a significant deterioration in the individual's functioning that this person is highly prone to a secondary condition such as pneumonia which becomes difficult to treat.]

THE PROGRESSION OF ALZHEIMER'S DISEASE

There are no two Alzheimer's victims the same! The location and amount of brain damage experienced varies from one person to another. This means that the symptoms and the level of functioning of one Alzheimer's victim may not be seen in another. This factor dictates that if there are no commonalties in symptoms there can be no universality in approach.

This lack of commonalty is the main problem encountered in caring for those who are mentally impaired versus caring for those who are physically disabled/cognitively well.

You are assigned to care for three stroke victims, each cognitively well with complete right sided paralysis. Although there may be a slight variation in their symptoms, there is considerable commonalty in their limitations. You can virtually establish a care process – appropriate approach, environment and programs – for one that will apply to all three.

The problem with three Alzheimer's victims is the lack of similarity in the symptoms presented. You can be assigned three Alzheimer's Victims – one has difficulty finding her room, but can remember faces; another has problems remembering faces, but can find her room; and the third can neither find her room nor remember faces. With such a variance in limitations, there can be little similarity in the care process – approach, environment and programs. What you establish for one will not be appropriate for the other two.

IT IS THE SYMPTOMS PRESENTED BY THE
INDIVIDUAL MENTALLY IMPAIRED RESIDENT THAT
DICTATES THE DIRECTION OF CARE.

Supportive Therapy is the key – identifying for that individual his strengths and maintaining them; identifying his limitations and compensating for them. Knowing that such an approach will be required for this person for the rest of his life and also knowing that his condition will worsen and further deteriorate given time. The goal of such an approach is to identify the person's maximum functioning level and maintain it. Holding an Alzheimer's victim at his existing level is a win. Curing him is an impossibility.

MULTIPLE INFARCT DISEASE

A second very common condition causing mental impairment in the elderly is Multiple Infarct Disease (MID). This condition is a series of small strokes due to a dysfunction in the circulatory system of the brain. The difference between Multiple Infarct Disease and what is commonly known as a "stroke", is the lack of physical paralysis. The damage experienced in MID usually causes a dysfunction in mental ability only and the symptoms presented very much resemble those commonly encountered with Alzheimer's disease. What differs between MID and Alzheimer's is the course and progression.

36

Unlike Alzheimer's disease, Multiple Infarct Disease can be very quick in its onset. When the individual experiences the first "stroke", obvious changes in cognitive functioning can be noticed.

Like any "stroke", the initial trauma or assault to the brain causes edema or swelling of brain tissue. This swelling can result in the victim demonstrating severe and multiple symptoms. As the swelling decreases over time, many of the initial symptoms may abate. You have seen individual's who have experienced total right sided paralysis regain much of their functioning within only a few weeks of experiencing the stroke. What may only remain is a flaccid or limp right arm. The same is true of Multiple Infarct Disease. The severity and multiplicity of the symptoms may improve somewhat after the initial onset.

The most significant issue with this disease is that when one cerebral infarct or "stroke" is encountered, the chances are high that in three days, three months or three years another may be experienced. This step-down deterioration – stroke, loss in functioning, slight improvement, stabilizing for a period, then stroke, loss of functioning, slight improvement, etc. – may continue until death (see diagram #2). Death is often caused by a major cerebral hemorrhage.

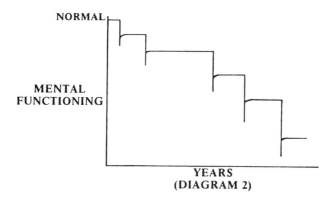

(DIAGRAM 2)

To demonstrate the course and progression of this condition, let us examine an actual case. We will call him John (age 69).

One Tuesday afternoon John sat in his favorite easy chair for a nap. When he woke half an hour later he was completely confused, disoriented and violent, striking out at family members who approached him. He was taken to hospital. Two weeks after his admission he improved considerably. His memory had returned, he was able to identify members of the family, he knew where he was.

The residual effect of the initial "stroke" was his inability to problem solve at a very basic level. From that point on, if you asked him to place a top on a pen he had considerable difficulty completing the task. He even had problems at times getting into a box of chocolates. All of his other faculties and abilities seemed to be functioning well.

The next month he experienced another cerebral infarct. It was very subtle; possibly showing itself as a slight dizzy spell or momentary blackout. It could even have happened during his sleep. Now he lost control over his emotions. He could not stop crying even though he expressed that he felt fine. The next month he had a major hemorrhage which finally did kill him.

The interventions employed in caring for an individual with Multiple Infarct Disease are the same as those for Alzheimer's – identify that person's strengths and maintain them, identify his limitations and compensate – Supportive Therapy.

PRIMARY TREATABLE CAUSES OF CONFUSION & DISORIENTATION

If all we were dealing with were chronic, irreversible conditions then our job would be much simpler. Mental dysfunctioning in the elderly can be caused by a multitude of conditions. Many of these causes can be treated and the originating symptoms reversed.

Let us examine a possible scenario:

Imagine:
>It is 1930
>You and I are married/
>We have five children/
>I work 12 hours per day at least 6 days a week
>At home I take care of all financial matters
>Do the repairs and house maintenance

Being the only one who drives, I do all the chauffeuring/
Your day consists mainly of household duties
Cooking, cleaning, raising the kids/

Our roles are distinct, not by choice but by necessity/
We find the only way to make ends meet is to divide the
        responsibility in what is needed to be done
Our dependency upon each other increases over time/

It is 1987/
I am retired and the kids are living on their own/
Who cooks?

> I help when needed, but I never had to learn to
> cook, you were always there. I can do a few things,
> but I never learned enough around the kitchen to do
> a complete meal.

Who cleans?

> You are 76 and I am 78. You went shopping for a
> few hours leaving me at home. On your return I
> greet you with "Hon I just cleaned the whole house
> for you from top to bottom". You know your
> definition of clean and mine are not the same and
> you will probably have to re-do it later. Another
> skill I did not have to master in our 56 years of
> marriage.

> I still take care of the repairs and maintenance of
> the house, the needed driving and all money
> matters including the bills/

I die/

What happens to you?

It is important to examine the impact of my loss on your life:

1. Depression – 56 of your 76 years have been spent with me. My
        loss creates in you a feeling of
        helplessness/hopelessness, an empty feeling that

has you questioning your own ability to put meaning into your life now that I am gone. The depression caused by the loss creates an apathy, a loss of energy and desire to do almost anything. You find little need to dress in the morning in anything other than a housecoat. Your involvement in almost everything grinds to a halt.

2. Isolation & Withdrawal – Being unable to drive, you find yourself virtually immobilized. This immobility and your desire to be left alone results in your spending much of your day in front of the television. At times it seems the only company you have is the TV. At least it breaks the silence.

3. Improper Diet – It becomes difficult to cook for one when you have been used to cooking for two or more for the past 56 years. You find little enjoyment in cooking now. Besides, your appetite doesn't seem to be like it was. Your meals now consist of mainly tea and toast or anything handy. Nibbling when and if you get hungry.

4. Over or under medicated – You become oblivious to time. You either forget to take your medication or you take too many – "It's 10 a.m. Did I take my 8 o'clock pill? I don't remember." You repeat the drug, doubling the dose.

5. Uncontrolled disease process – Taking your medication at irregular times, if taking it at all, results in any existing physical problem worsening and your health deteriorating.

Six months pass!
You are very ill/
Mentally you appear confused and disoriented/
You are admitted to hospital with the following problems:

Depression,
Electrolyte Imbalance,

Dehydration,
Over or Under Medicated,
A Pre–existing Disease Process Out of Control

While in hospital
Your physical and mental state return to near normal/

The factors contributing to this turn–around are simple – you are in contact with others, encouraged to eat and dress, your medication is controlled – other than the loss of your husband and your depression, everything that caused the symptoms has been removed.

On admission to hospital, you will have mimicked many of the symptoms associated with Alzheimer's disease. This scenario is a typical example demonstrating the process of Primary Causes of Confusion & Disorientation – a condition that creates a symptomology resembling Alzheimer's or other related disorders but is treatable (in years past called Acute Organic Brain Syndrome).

There are a large number of causes of confusion and disorientation in the elderly. Here is but a brief list:

Hypoxia	Drug Related Intoxications
Anemia	Pernicious Anemia
Nutritional Deficiencies	Pellagara
Cardiac Decompensation	Stress
Hypotension	Increased Intracranial Pressure
Hypothyroidism	Sensory Deprivation
Respiratory Disease	Depression
Myocardial Infarction	Anxiety
Dehydration	Pain
Electrolyte Imbalance	Systemic Infection
Hyper/Hypocalcemia	Hearing or Visual Loss
Endocrine Dysfunction	Environmental Changes
Hypo/hyperthermia	Loneliness

The risk of these conditions being easily misdiagnosed as an irreversible organic brain syndrome in the elderly can be high, given the right circumstances.

A few years ago a 66 year old man was admitted from an acute care facility to a unit for the mentally impaired. The diagnosis received on his transfer was Alzheimer's disease. His wife (62 years of age) was no longer able to care for him at home. His increasing dependency on her and his periodic violent outbursts created a 24 hour per day job that exhausted her.

On admission to the long term care facility, she stated that his condition developed only 6 months earlier. From the onset until now it had gotten progressively worse.

The long term care facility in which he was admitted had a well functioning unit for the mentally impaired. A short time after admission his case was reviewed. The staff working on the unit felt this man did not match the "picture" normally encountered with other residents diagnosed as suffering from Alzheimer's disease, yet they could not identify specifically what was different.

As his case was discussed, the head nurse of the unit recalled a similar case a few years earlier. At that time an older man living on the unit demonstrated similar symptoms and behaviours – confusion, disorientation, violent outbursts. Many factors in this older resident's case were reviewed. At one point the team began to experiment with his medications knowing he had a high sensitivity to a number of drugs in the past. When a specific anti–hypertensive drug was changed to another, his violent outbursts stopped. He was still confused and disoriented, but no longer aggressive. It was believed that he experienced an allergic reaction to that specific anti–hypertensive agent and this reaction caused his violent outbursts.

This 66 year old resident the team was now discussing was on the same anti–hypertensive medication. The doctor agreed to try this man on another drug. His anti–hypertensive agent was changed. In three weeks the man was off the unit and in three months he was back home and perfectly normal. It was believed that he experienced a toxic or an allergic reaction to the drug, which caused his confusion, disorientation and violent outbursts.

You may question how this can be allowed to happen. The answer relates to what was discussed in chapter one – the outcome depends on the aggressiveness of the assessment undertaken at the time of diagnosis. Any of the treatable causes of confusion and disorientation can result in an older person looking and acting the same as an Alzheimer's victim. The person's mental functioning level will deteriorate over time but at a certain point stabilize, holding at a specific level for a considerable period (see diagram #3 solid line). If the cause of this acute bout of confusion and disorientation is eliminated, the person will return to his normal functioning level (dotted line).

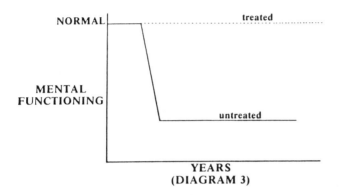

(DIAGRAM 3)

The dilemma we face in dealing with many reversible causes of mental impairment is that the longer there is a lack of treatment the greater the chances that the condition may become impossible to reverse.

The chances of a misdiagnosis of Alzheimer's disease in some situations can be high. As mentioned earlier, there are only two ways to diagnosis Alzheimer's – through a process of elimination or by an autopsy after death. If a thorough assessment has not been completed on any resident at the time of diagnosing, then how is it known that we are dealing with Alzheimer's and not something treatable?

A basic work up to determine the presence of treatable factors causing mental impairment in the elderly includes the following:

CBC (Complete Blood Count)	Stool for Occult Blood
T_3T_4	Urinalysis/Culture
Calcium	Syphilis
B_{12}	Chest X-ray

43

Sedimentation Rate
Electrolytes   EKG (Electrocardiogram)
Phosphorous   Rectal, Pelvic, Neurological
BUN (Blood Urea Nitrogen)   Exam
Blood Sugar   Drug Toxicity Level
Liver Function   Psychological Assessment

This battery of tests needs to be initiated on any older person showing a change in cognitive functioning. The fact that such a work-up would be commonplace for any person under 65 showing signs of confusion, disorientation and a decrease in cognitive functioning makes it mandatory for all over 65.

SUMMARY

You will have heard of other conditions causing mental impairment (Pick's Disease for example), but these so closely resemble Alzheimer's in course and progression that it is not significant to isolate them in our discussion. Often the difference between Alzheimer's and these other conditions can only be noted at the time of autopsy when brain tissue is examined microscopically.

Rather than investing further energies to expand the biological nature of the disease process, it is more important to identify what we as caregivers can do to assist the mentally impaired to live to their fullest. Many believe after learning about Alzheimer's and Multiple Infarct Disease that little can be done. On the contrary, much can be done. Curing or reversing the organic changes experienced by the brain is not possible, but providing the victims of such disorders the highest level of quality of life given the circumstances experienced is our main responsibility.

To determine the most appropriate living environment for any mentally impaired resident requires that we define this person's vulnerability. The mentally impaired are sensitive to the world around them. Any mentally impaired resident may experience further limitations in his functioning ability by external factors including inappropriate approach, an underlying disease process, a faulty drug profile and a confusing environment. Much can be done on our part to control each of these situations in order for each resident to achieve his highest level of quality of life given his limitations.

Chapter Three

Secondary Factors

[A Reminder – the remaining portions of this text will discuss those mentally impaired who are at level two functioning ability as described in Chapter Two. These are the most challenging. Any concepts presented that are effective with this group, can easily be adapted for level one and three.]

The sensitivity of the mentally impaired residents to external factors is a major concern for the caregiver. Secondary factors are external circumstances that further impair the functioning ability of an individual with Alzheimer's or Multiple Infarct disease.

This sensitivity can be divided into four categories:
1. Drugs
2. Disease
3. Approach
4. Environment

If any of these factors are not controlled, the cognitive ability of a mentally impaired resident will decrease, resulting in an increase in inappropriate behaviour, be it apathy or agitation. Diagram #4 demonstrates the potential change that can occur in a person's functioning level. The course of the disease is the dotted line. The sudden drop in the person's mental functioning level (solid line) can be the result of one of the above factors.

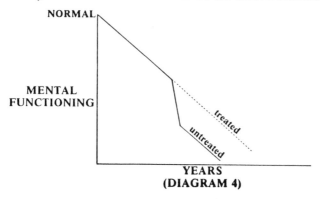

(DIAGRAM 4)

DRUGS

The sensitivity of older people to medication has been a long standing concern. Aging creates specific biological changes that can alter bodily functions. These changes have the ability to effect the older person's response to many medications. Some of the major physical aging changes that can affect drug utilization are:

- a decrease in effective absorption of substances through the gastrointestinal tract
- a slowing of metabolism or the breakdown of substances within the body
- less effective excretion of substances from the body
- alterations in the circulatory system in transporting substances within the body
- changes in the location and amount of fat deposits affecting the storage of substances within the body

The majority of these changes are gradual in nature and usually moderate in their degree. As a result, most older people do not experience from these changes any restrictions in their ability to function in their daily living activities. However, it is apparent that these changes can effect medication use by increasing the risk of a toxic level of even therapeutic drugs.

The following is a brief list of some of the commonly used therapeutic medications that can cause confusion and disorientation in the elderly.

Antihypertensive Agents		Antidepressant Agents
Aldactazide	Hydropes	Elavil
Aldactone	Inderal	Etrafon
Aldomet	Rauzide	Sinequan
Aldoril	Regroton	Tofranil
Apresoline	Ser–Ap–Es	Triavil
Diupres		

Antiarthritic Agents	Antianxiety Agents
Butazolidin	Librium
Indocin	Meprobamate
Tandearil	Serax
	Tranxene
	Valium

Others

Ambenyl Expectorant for cough	Gantanol for infection
Azo Gantrisin for urinary tract infection	Koan for potassium depletion
	Librax for relief of gastrointestinal symptoms
Benadryl for allergies	
Dalmane for sleep	Lomotil for diarrhea
Demerol for pain	Mellaril for psychiatric disorders
Dilantin for epilepsy	Periactin for allergies
Dimetane for allergy	Tigan for nausea and vomiting
Drixoral for nasal decongestant	

Determining the most effective drug to treat a specific disorder experienced by an older person is not an easy process. What complicates it further is that the physical changes caused by the aging process happen at different times, to a different intensity with each person. It is then difficult to predict whether a medication taken by one older person would have the same impact on another. Toxic or adverse effects experienced by one older person to a specific drug does not mean that another will not be able to tolerate and benefit from that same medication.

This individuality in drug response is characteristic to the mentally impaired as well. Some medications work well with certain mentally impaired residents, while those same drugs at the same dosage have a devastating effect on others.

These discrepancies are complicated even further by the fact that the mentally impaired are significantly more sensitive to medication than the older population in general. This makes medication use with the mentally impaired a major concern.

The information on medication use and the elderly is growing, but information on medication effects on the mentally impaired elderly is limited. This lack of information makes it difficult to discuss specific brand name drugs when talking about their potential impact on the mentally impaired. In our discussion, specific examples can only refer to categories of medications rather than brand names themselves. Besides, it is not the specific drug that is important but understanding the impact of any medication on any one mentally impaired person that is the issue. With any mentally impaired resident, functioning on all counts can deteriorate dramatically given the wrong medication at the wrong time.

Sleeping medications or hypnotics are prime examples of this phenomenon. Certain sleeping pills have a devastating effect on the mentally impaired. One popular drug in this category has what is called a "100 hour half life" in some individuals over 65. (half life is the length of time it takes for half of one dose to be excreted from the body.) In simpler terms this means if I am 78, and sensitive to that specific drug, once administered it will take 100 hours for half of one dose to leave my body. Give me that same pill five nights in a row. The effect? The same impact as our discussion on Demerol in chapter one.

Give this same sleeping pill to a mentally impaired individual who is as sensitive. Administer it to him five nights in a row. Then place his breakfast in front of him on the sixth morning. The result? He will be unable to feed himself.

This change in functioning ability has nothing to do directly with the disease process experienced but totally to his sensitivity to this secondary factor (diagram #4).

A similar effect can be encountered with almost every category of medication. Antianxiety agents are another example. Certain commonly used drugs in this group have a half life equivalent to age. This means if I am 80 years old and sensitive to this specific medication, it will take 80 hours for half of that drug to leave my body once administered. Some of these agents possess a 6 half life duration (the entire length of time for the drug to be totally eliminated from the body) – if I take that drug now, it takes 6 times 80 or 480 hours, twenty days for all of that drug to leave my body (the first 80 hours, half of the dose leaves my body, the second 80 hours, half of the half, etc.). Give me that medication three times a day for a month. The result is a highly and even toxic sedating affect, decreasing the person's ability to concentrate and perform at many tasks.

The negative impact of certain medications on the elderly can be dramatic. We know little about the effect of one drug on an older person let alone a combination of possibly 5, 8 or 10 different medications taken in a 24 hour period. This sensitivity is compounded even further with the mentally impaired elderly. Their reaction to any one drug may be as great as four times what is experienced by the older population in general. This makes medication use with the mentally impaired elderly a primary concern.

Whenever a mentally impaired resident's behaviour changes or functioning level deteriorates (whether physically, mentally or emotionally) the first questions that must be asked are:

What change has been made to the dose or times of
medications given?
What new drug has been ordered?

If a recent change in medication has occurred, then that is the first area to be investigated as its possible cause.

The sensitivity of any mentally impaired older person to medication creates the need for ongoing assessment and a conscious trial and error approach in medication usage – starting an older person on a specific medication, observing closely for side effects created, being willing to alter the type or dose of the drug should side effects persist.

In fact, the best philosophy with medication use and the mentally impaired elderly is – "When in doubt, do without".

DRUGS – WHEN IN DOUBT
DO WITHOUT

Chapter eleven will discuss the process of medication assessments and usage in detail.

DISEASE

If a mentally impaired resident experiences a bout of the flu – diarrhea or upper respiratory tract infection, what is the effect on his mental state? In many cases his mental function will decrease, his confusion and disorientation will increase (a drop in functioning as noted in diagram #4).

Any acute or chronic disease process can have the same results. A mentally impaired individual experiencing congestive heart failure which is usually controlled by medication, encounters an acute episode of that condition – short of breath, diaphoretic (severe sweating), cyanotic (bluish colouration of the skin), etc. During that time and even for some time after he is restabilized, there will be an obvious decline in his cognitive level. The acute episode effected blood flow to the brain, as well as creating increased stress on all organs of the body, thereby decreasing the brain's performance, and potentially increasing the level of confusion experienced.

The organic changes experienced by the brain of a person with Alzheimer's or Multiple Infarct Disease can create considerable sensitivity to alterations in any body process. The brain's effectiveness to perform can be hampered by changes to any of the major organs of the body – liver, heart, lungs, circulatory system, kidneys, etc.

The successful treatment of this secondary disease (flu, acute bout of congestive heart failure, etc.) will usually result in a return of the person's functioning level to its original state (the level before the onset of that treatable condition).

A person having Alzheimer's or Multiple Infarct Disease has no increased immunity against the ailments and afflictions suffered by the population in general. In fact the mentally impaired individual may be significantly more sensitive to these factors than the population at large. Medical assessment and intervention are as essential to the well-being of the mentally impaired as to anyone else. If aggressive medical assessment and intervention is not a significant facet of the care process, then achieving the desired level of quality of life for the mentally impaired becomes an impossibility.

Ongoing medical assessment is the key to ensure that any further changes in cognitive functioning is directly related to Alzheimer's or Multiple Infarct disease and is not the result of a treatable secondary disease process. A basic medical assessment must be part of the assessment process. Such an assessment must be completed on admission, during the yearly medical, and whenever a change is noted.

A basic medical work-up as a normal part of the assessment process ensures that the degree of limitation experienced by any resident has been thoroughly examined medically to establish that the cause is not one that could be easily rectified by a simple medical intervention of a specific medication, diet, etc.

Medical investigation does not stop because a person has the diagnosis of Alzheimer's or Multiple Infarct Disease. It is essential that the physician in charge of this resident still investigates for treatable factors should the symptoms merit it.

Rationalizing changes in functioning ability or behaviour to the original diagnosis without adequate assessment is a narrow and dangerous route to take. The right of the mentally impaired to be well is no different than the right of all of us.

It is equally as important to conserve the time and energies of the care team as well. To introduce programming to compensate for something that can easily be treated medically (infection, diabetes, etc.) is senseless. When working with the mentally impaired, external factors must be ruled out before any other long term interventions are employed.

APPROACH

Chapter two presented the following scenario:

> You are mentally impaired
> Sitting in your chair/
> At 0845 hours I enter your room
> To take you to the bathroom/
> Standing over you I ask "Do you have to go to the
>   washroom?"/
> Without any further direction
> I take you by the elbow to assist you to stand
> You resist, becoming aggressive and defensive/

The mentally impaired resident may experience a chronic emotional state of anxiety and fear. With the inability to analyze situations and events, all one can do is read the actions and behaviours of others at face value. This makes a person highly prone to eliciting a defensive response to any situation that is not clearly understood. Taking you by the elbow and making you stand without much warning creates a very threatening experience. Being unable to remember who I am or where you are, you cannot determine where I am taking you. My actions as you see them, justifies only one logical response – to become defensive in order to protect yourself.

If the agitation created by this event ended when you left the room, there would be little problem. That is not always the case. Instead it is more common that the heightened level of fear and anxiety will remain. With some residents it can last for hours, with others the rest of the day.

In fact, this heightened fear and anxiety could spill over to other staff, situations and other shifts. That one event could effect the success of any staff. During that day, even those who normally have little difficulty taking you to the washroom, may now find you difficult to handle.

Once the anxiety level of the mentally impaired resident is increased, it may take some time for a sense of security to return. During this heightened anxiety there exists a strong suspicious tendency when interpreting the actions of others. Normal tasks and performance levels will be dramatically affected during this period (diagram #4).

This effect can be demonstrated further. If I approached you at 1130 hours in the manner described above, causing you to become agitated, what would be your response when I place your lunch in front of you at 1130 hours? I would hope that I have another clean uniform; I may be wearing your lunch.

You know well the effects of a staff member who employs an inappropriate approach when caring for the mentally impaired. If you can arrive on duty at 7 in the morning and know exactly who was working the previous night shift by the number of mentally impaired residents who are agitated and/or wandering then you have identified the effect. The change in a resident's behaviour is often due to the elevated anxiety created by the approach and environment encountered. Once one's anxiety level is increased, mental functioning deteriorates. The resident is now unable to perform tasks he could easily perform under more supportive circumstances.

ENVIRONMENT

A team of professionals visited a 30 bed unit for the mentally impaired elderly. Initially they found the majority of residents sitting. They saw little wandering and no agitated behaviour. After 10 minutes of their walking about the unit, talking to staff and amongst themselves, there was a noted increase in wandering and aggressive behaviour of the residents.

If a stimulus in the environment cannot easily be identified or clarified by the mentally impaired, it increases anxiety. An increase in anxiety decreases mental functioning, thereby increasing wandering or agitated behaviour.

This is an important concept – anyone in contact with the mentally impaired can influence care. Initially when I was on one unit for the mentally impaired, the majority of residents were sitting quietly in the lounge apparently listening to music from the stereo. There was little wandering or aggressive behaviour seen anywhere at this time. The head nurse and I were standing in the hall talking when a maintenance man carrying an aluminum ladder walked onto the unit. He erected the ladder in front of the lounge door and began tearing tile from the ceiling and shouting to another maintenance man down the hall. Within a short time a number of the mentally impaired residents who were in the lounge became restless and some began wandering. Finally the agitated behaviour of other residents in the lounge disrupted the music session.

The residents in the lounge did not understand the noise or where it originated. All they knew was that they heard a noise they could not comprehend. This unknown stimulus increased their anxiety, causing some to wander and others to become agitated.

Previous to that incident many of the residents in the lounge were able to listen to the music. Once the environment intensified their anxiety, the mental functioning of some to concentrate on that task decreased. As a result, a task that normally could be performed was now severely curtailed. (see diagram #4)

Is there a difference in the activity and noise level on your unit at 1000 hours on Sunday morning compared to 0900 hours Monday morning? If your response is "yes", then you have just authenticated the potential effects of an uncontrolled environment.

While assessing one unit, I stood at what was known as the crossroads (a hall to my back, one to my front and one to the left and right). It was 1000 hours on a Monday morning. Located in the corner in front of me and to my left was an open lounge. In that lounge the TV and the radio were on at the same time. Two very confused residents were talking to themselves quite loudly. Another resident was yelling to be allowed out of the chair. At the opposite corner was the nurse's station. The doctor and nurse were talking about orders. The phone was ringing. Behind me coming up the hall was another resident being pushed in a wheelchair. It was time for her bath, and it was definite she didn't want a bath given the commotion she demonstrated. Above me announcements were heard over the PA system. In front of me a housekeeper was running the floor polisher. Imagine the state and functioning ability of the level two mentally impaired on that unit at that time. The problem created, remained even after the noise level had subsided. In fact, in this situation the effects of the bombarding lasted for hours. The agitation and confusion level of many of the residents was elevated and their ability to function decreased for some time afterwards.

Each of these factors: drugs, disease, approach and environment can dramatically effect the success of any mentally impaired residents to survive in our environment. Some say there is little that can be done with the mentally impaired. Given what has just been presented, it is easy to reveal the sensitivity of the mentally impaired. As a result, their need for a controlled, supportive environment demonstrates that there is much that can be done. However, it does not end there. There are more, not so obvious issues that can have a significant impact on the lives of the mentally impaired. Let us examine them to some depth.

THE EFFECTS OF LABELING

All of us have experienced the effects of labeling. There is probably no one in any work environment who has not been labeled, at one time or another. If you are labeled a "_ _ _ _ disturber" (you fill in the blank), then all you have to do in a meeting or conversation is raise your concerns and immediately someone around you will comment "Here she goes again!"

Labeling effects how we perceive an individual and subsequently how we treat that person. If staff identify the director of nursing as a "tyrant" or "holy terror", then that belief will contaminate any contact they have with that person, influencing their response and expectations of the outcome. Going to that person's office to make a simple request sets staff quivering, with an expectation that the request will be denied. What demonstrates the intensity and effects of a label and its effects is when the opposite of what is expected is encountered. Let me show you.

Imagine the scenario unfolding as follows:

55

You approach my office door to make your request/
Your expectation is that I will be resistive
And probably say "no"./
You knock on my door
I open it saying
"Hi, how are you? Come on in."/
I ask you to sit in one of my comfortable lounge chairs in
       the corner/
"Can I get you a coffee?"
"How's the family?"
We talk about your family for 10 minutes/
"What can I do for you?"
You make your request.
You don't get exactly what you want
Instead you get a compromise you are very pleased with/
You return to the unit/
As soon as the other staff see you they ask
"How did it go?"/
You respond "Great!
He asked me into my office
Sat me into his comfortable chair
Talked about my family
Got me a cup of coffee
And gave me almost everything that I wanted!"/

There is no question that the response by some staff who only see that boss through the label of being a "tyrant" would be "What's he want? What's he after?" Labels are powerful. They make unpredictable behaviour predictable. Something that <u>could</u> happen is expected to occur <u>every</u> time, in <u>every</u> situation. In the above scenario, staff expected a difficult and abrasive response from the manager, when it was not received they tried to second guess the motive behind the change. They are always looking to justify the label, any change from what was "expected" met with suspicion and was believed to be out of character.

Imagine:

      I am mentally impaired
      Living in a long term care facility
      Often confused and disoriented/

> Who places me in front of my closet to pick my own
> clothes?

Staff or family who function by labeling behaviour may have an expectation that when a person is confused and disoriented about many things around him, then he is probably confused about most, if not all things. As a result, no one with such a restrictive viewpoint would place that person in front of his closet, believing it would be a waste of time, even though the person may have the ability to pick some of his clothing.

You are a new staff member to the unit. You work with this mentally impaired resident for a couple of days and complete your own assessment.

> Through your observations
> You believe I am capable of picking my own clothes/
> So you place me in front of my closet to pick my clothes
> For the first time in months/

What happens?

Probably nothing! This resident would stand in front of the closet and make little or no attempt to pick out any clothing.

The definition of Supportive Therapy stated – identify the individual's limitations and compensate for them; identify the person's strengths and maintain them. In caring for the mentally impaired the second statement is as important as the first. When a strength or ability of a mentally impaired resident is neglected or over–looked, and then he is asked to perform at a much later date, there is a good chance he will not be as successful as he once was. Whether that task is eating, dressing, shaving, picking clothes or communicating, the impact of inactivity for the mentally impaired remains the same – "If you don't use it, you lose it!"

When a mentally impaired resident is not encouraged to maintain existing strengths, he will undoubtedly lose the ability to perform as well as before. Re–learning the task at a later date is hampered by his cognitive impairment. The probability of his regaining that original level of functioning is reduced. As a result, his competency level will deteriorate simply because of the expectations of others.

I was counselling a resident in a semi–private room. My client was unavoidably called away for 15 minutes during the session. I decided to take this opportunity to meet her roommate. Her roommate was well over 90 years old, weighed about 65 pounds and was in a frozen fetal position due to long standing muscle contractures.

Before approaching any resident, I will always check with staff if there is information I need to know about that person (hearing problem, speech difficulty, cognitive dysfunction, etc.) in order to adjust my approach appropriately. When I asked staff about my client's roommate, I was told by one staff member "Don't even bother talking to that lady, she is so confused she won't even answer."

Such a comment initiates an immediate response on my part as I know it does with you – the need to confirm such an absolute before determining what can and cannot be done. I approached my client's roommate. She was lying in bed, where she spent much of her time. While in bed she could lie in only one of two positions – left side or right side. I squatted down, placed my face close to hers and asked "How are you?" She said "Fine!"

In my conversation with this lady, I found she had a sense of humour that would "knock your socks off". Throughout our conversation she would lose track of what we were discussing and go off on a tangent, but it was easy to draw her back on topic.

In examining a situation such as this, it is of little value to define right or wrong. It is more important to determine what is happening and how to change it. The circumstances that seemed to lead to the label of "confused – will not communicate" were straightforward. Often care was performed by two staff at one time – one to hold and assist with turning and moving, while the other performed the needed tasks. A bed bath and back rub was completed in the following manner: the resident was placed on her right side, a staff member stood at the one side of her bed holding her over, the other staff member stood at the other side washing and rubbing her back. During the procedure, the conversation was mainly between the two staff. Every once in awhile one of the staff would look down at this resident and ask "What do you think about that Mrs. Brown?" All Mrs. Brown could see was the caregiver's waist (when the stimulus is not intense enough, it will be missed or misinterpreted). She did not know who they were talking to or even possibly what they were saying, so she did not answer.

This scenario need only be repeated a few times until Mrs. Brown's lack of response was labeled as confused. Based on their contact and their interaction with her, staff believed she was incapable of communicating coherently when asked a question. Once the label was established, few staff believed it worthwhile to go into her room and talk with her when she was sitting quietly. In this case, a lady who had the ability to communicate was restricted due to the inappropriate and limiting expectations of those around her. The longer she was restricted in her contact with others, the greater the chance her communicative skills would deteriorate because of her limited interaction with others. Over time it would become harder and harder for her to maintain a conversation thereby fulfilling the label – "confused".

Any label can present the same dimensions – confused, dirty old man, aggressive, etc. The impact of any label makes unpredictable behaviour predictable. Setting an expectation of a person below his existing ability and providing no other option to allow the person to meet his potential.

Being labeled aggressive creates a similar phenomenon. A mentally impaired resident who was considered "aggressive" was approached by two staff to give him his shave. While the man was sitting quietly in his chair in the lounge, the two staff stood in front of him about five feet away and looking down at him said "Mr. Giovanni it's time for your shave!" One of the staff walked around to his left side and slightly behind him, the other walked around to his right. Their next actions almost seemed choreographed, both staff simultaneously placed one hand on the resident's shoulder and with their other hands, grabbed each of the man's wrists. Mr. Giovanni began struggling.

I asked the staff why he was approached in that manner. Their response was "He always fights when he has to have a shave, I'm not about to let him kick me." I then asked how they would have approached him had he not been labeled "aggressive". One stated she would have brought the razor with her (they normally didn't bring the razor fearing if he saw it he would become aggressive immediately); she would kneel next to him; touch him to get his attention; show him the razor; pantomime the actions of shaving and gently guide him out of the chair.

Their initial approach of grabbing him while he sat in the chair gave Mr. Giovanni no option but to defend himself. The more he responded to their actions in this manner, the more he reinforced their belief of his "being aggressive", further justifying their approach.

Not only was Mr. Giovanni aggressive during this one encounter, but the agitation initiated during his shave lingered for hours. Once his anxiety level was elevated, he had considerable difficulty functioning at any task – he was unable to sit for any length of time, unable to eat without being easily distracted, unable to concentrate on any activities he could perform when his anxiety level was lower. Each aggressive outburst only intensified the label until it was expected by many staff that every encounter with him would lead to an aggressive response.

The scenario in chapter two further exemplifies this. I approached you in your room at 0845 hours to take you to the bathroom, standing over you and looking down I asked you if you "have to go". When you did not answer, I took you out of the chair with little warning. Your response was naturally to resist and become aggressive. If after the toileting fiasco, I approached other staff and said "Watch out, she tried to kick me in a place I don't want to mention." Few would enter your room and stand in front of you. Most would approach you from behind, always standing to your side or back. If you had any suspicion before, it would only be intensified now. Your potential for an aggressive outburst will increase with each encounter.

Labels can be deadly! The staff who have the greatest tendency to label resident's behaviour are those who have the most difficulty with the mentally impaired. Often these staff are structured in their routine and see much of the behaviour of the mentally impaired as being subjective, believing the resident is capable of controlling it if he wanted. Those staff who can relate to the mentally impaired have a better understanding of the circumstances leading to a resident's response and are more apt to adjust their approach and care based on what the resident needs at that time.

Describing behaviour as aggressive, confused, etc. is appropriate. It indicates to staff what may happen, whereas the label sets an expectation that on every contact it <u>will</u> happen. The most important thing in dealing with any behaviour or ability of the mentally impaired is to "check it out". What was encountered yesterday with that person by certain staff does not mean it will be encountered today by you.

SUMMARY

The mentally impaired elderly are highly sensitive to the things around them. Almost anything has the ability to effect their cognitive level and behaviour. Any lack on the caregiver's part to be sensitive to these issues and constantly attempt to control them, will have a major detrimental effect on their effectiveness and the subsequent quality of life of those under their care.

What has and will be continually emphasized throughout this text is the individuality and uniqueness of each person suffering from mental impairment. Certain aspects of approach, environment, drugs and disease may have a major impact on one person; less of an effect on another and no negative effects on a third.

This uniqueness of response can be demonstrated with no more clarity than when we examine the variety of symptoms associated with the disease.

Chapter Four

Symptoms of Mental Impairment

The symptoms associated with mental impairment are varied and complex. There are virtually no two residents with the same in the combination of symptoms, behaviours and degree of loss in functioning ability. Such a variance emphasizes the importance of assessment. Until the individual's strengths and limitations are defined, care direction cannot be accurately determined.

When discussing some of the following symptoms, specific assessment mechanisms and guidelines on appropriate programming will also be presented. Further details of specific intervention strategies will be further expanded in subsequent chapters.

JUDGMENT

Impairment to judgment represents a loss in the ability to differentiate extremes – the differences between right/wrong; good/bad; too much/too little. When an individual with this limitation is placed in front of a closet to pick out his own clothes, he will put on three pairs of pants and two shirts. Similarly, if a resident is given her make-up, she will undoubtedly become bizarre in appearance, not knowing when to stop. Giving a certain resident his breakfast may result in his pouring coffee into his cereal. A person with an impairment in judgment only knows that something has to be done, so he does it. He cannot define limits or determine the consequences of many of his actions.

Usually this person is not aware of there being a problem. In fact, it appears that those with an impairment in judgment are often pleased with what they have accomplished. Not being able to identify any limits to their actions, they are unable to identify when they have gone too far, believing they have done the task appropriately. To corroborate this, watch how a female Alzheimer's victim responds to her attempt at applying make-up. Even though she is bizarre in her appearance, she acts as though everything is fine.

Constantly correcting this individual is often not effective and may even lead to an aggressive response. The aggressiveness is due to the obvious conflict of you seeing something wrong when the resident feels everything is fine. To say to this person "Look what you have done to your face", creates a state of confusion. When challenged in such a manner, she becomes confused by the comment. As far as she is concerned there is nothing wrong with "her face". This confusion increases her anxiety level, creating the feeling of being out of control and resulting in an aggressive response.

In keeping with the mandate of Supportive Therapy – compensating for weaknesses and maintaining strengths – it is important to focus on what she has accomplished, rather than what she has not. To reprimand her for her action, when she is not aware that her action is inappropriate, will have a detrimental effect. Only minutes after the confrontation, she will probably not remember what was said about her make-up (due to her recent memory loss), but she will retain the emotions that were stirred from the comment. Subsequently her aggressive behaviour could last for hours afterwards.

The more effective approach is to focus on strengths, not limitations. In this scenario, her strength is obvious – she attempted to put on her make-up even though she has limited functioning ability. "Mary, you put on your make-up today, good for you. You missed a spot on your cheek with some of your blush. Why don't we go into your room and fix that and you'll look just great." This supportive response will likely result in her returning to her room more willingly than by confronting her with what she has done poorly.

Probably the most effective intervention in this situation is one that can be called anticipation. Anticipation is the process of defining a person's pattern of behaviour and then responding accordingly. This allows the caregiver to be prepared that at any time with any mentally impaired resident, there will be something out of place, something that needs to be corrected. If this lady has applied her (or someone else's make-up) four times in a row and has become bizarre in her appearance each time, then chances are high that the next time she has her hands on some make-up she will look the same. Anticipation does not solve the problem, it just removes the shock, preparing one for what might occur, setting in place a reaction that is appropriate to the person's limitations. For a staff member to respond "I told you the last time not to do that with your make-up" is not only a wasted effort but can cause a detrimental effect. First, she does not remember "the last time" and second, she is not aware that there is a problem now. Again she will forget what was said, but retain the emotions generated.

The most effective means of determining a resident's limitation in judgment involves frequent contact and observation. By identifying specific patterns in behaviour, one can also identify the interventions needed. This ongoing assessment becomes the key to successfully caring for the mentally impaired. Bizarre appearance in applying make-up requires someone to guide the resident through the process, setting the framework for a very appropriate activity program on a daily basis. The person who has difficulty combining clothes, will need them laid out on the bed to decrease the choices required. The resident who has problems with meal times requires staff to guide him in preparing his cereal or coffee. The 24 Hour Profile (discussed in chapter eleven) will assist in identifying any such patterns in behaviour and functioning.

ORIENTATION

Impairment in orientation will effect a mentally impaired person's ability to relate to either time, person, place or thing.

a) Time
Time is meaningless to many of those who are mentally impaired. The person's loss of recent memory makes it difficult to keep track of the time, day, month or year.

Knowing the time requires a person to be able to remember at least one point of reference. If today is Monday, then tomorrow is Tuesday. But if I cannot remember what is just told to me, then that point of reference is gone. Time is virtually lost. It becomes impossible for the mentally impaired resident to keep track of time for the simple fact that it is always changing. The more severe the person's impairment, the more difficulty in identifying time – some mentally impaired know the day, but not the time of day; others know the month but not the day, others only the year and still others nothing at all.

Being unable to identify the passage of time makes it difficult to keep track of the simple progression of hours in the day. Breakfast, lunch, supper, bedtime, awakening, bathing now have no reference point. This may result in the resident being spontaneous in his actions. Waking in the early hours of the morning, insisting it is time for breakfast; resisting going to meals, saying he just ate; not wanting a bath, believing he just had one, etc.

This disorientation requires all staff to constantly reinforce the "time" element when making contact. An expectation that the resident knows the time of day, let alone the day, can result in considerable resistance. We become the resident's "time piece".

Assessment:
What day is it today?
What month?
What year?

The response to these questions is significant to the caregiver in possibly understanding some of the behaviours of certain mentally impaired residents. Knowing the resident's time frame may explain the behaviours demonstrated (expanded further in the discussion of memory loss).

Clocks may be valuable to some mentally impaired, but the location and number on the unit is critical – the size and where the clock is placed will determine if it is used. A clock high on the wall, above eye level will never be seen. One that is small becomes invisible. Modern digital clocks are of little value to many mentally impaired – seeing the time as 0815 hours is meaningless.

The clock must be a large faced clock, with large numbers and hands, located at eye level on a wall that makes it visible from any point in the room. Before any resident is encouraged to read and use a clock, he must be assessed to determine if he can relate to one. To some mentally impaired, looking at even a large faced clock at eye level may provide as much information as looking at a blank wall.

Assessment:

>Place a clock in front of the resident and ask him to
>identify specified times.
>Place the hands of the clock at specific times (8, 12 and 5
>o'clock) and ask what would happen at those times
>(breakfast, lunch and supper).

If he is able to read and understand a clock placed in front of him,
then he may be able to use one in his room and in the lounge. If
he can identify key times of the day – 8 a.m., 12 noon, 5 p.m., 9
p.m., then he can be provided a schedule of his day in large, bold
print identifying breakfast, lunch, supper and bedtime. A clock on
its own may be of little value; a clock next to an event board can
be useful.

```
+-----------------------------------------------+
|  EVENT BOARD                                  |
|  8:00 a.m.     Breakfast                       |
|  12 Noon       Lunch      < NEXT |             |
|  5:00 p.m.     Supper                          |
|  8:00 p.m.     Bedtime                         |
+-----------------------------------------------+
```

Depending on the resident's functioning level, the event
board becomes an important reference to identify the next
activity. As one event is completed, the arrow (next) is moved
down. The clock next to the event board assists the resident to
determine how long before the next activity. Even if a person is
unable to relate to the clock, the sign itself may be of assistance.
Spaces are left on the event board after each main function to
insert the times of other events for that day (i.e. 10 a.m. –
exercises).

The most successful clock placed in the resident's lounge
is an old fashioned pendulum chime clock. The intention for this
device is not to assist the person in telling time, but to hook "old
memories". The chimes will attract the attention of many
residents to look at the clock potentially eliciting many old
memories, providing some interesting conversations.

The importance of constantly reinforcing time to the
mentally impaired must be questioned. A popular seminar that I

present is called "Does It Really Matter If Its Tuesday?" At the end of the session, participants would ask "Does it matter if its Tuesday to the mentally impaired?" My response was always the same "If I forget, you'll remember."

The reality is that few low functioning mentally impaired residents will be able to relate to such complex objects as clocks, event boards and calendars. That leaves staff as the main vehicle to provide the needed information – the time of the day. Telling the resident the day and time does not ensure that he will remember, but ensures the environment in which he lives attempts to compensate for the limitations he experiences.

b) Place

Impairment in recent memory makes it extremely difficult for a resident to remember where he is.

Assessment:

Where are you living now?
Is this where you work, a hospital, a nursing home or your
home?

The inability to respond correctly to the first question initiates the interviewer to ask the second.

The response to these questions provides significant information. Determining where the resident believes he is may explain some of the behaviours demonstrated and provide direction on the best course of action to be taken. A need to clean if it is believed to be home; an insistence of going home if it is believed to be work; soon to go home if believed to be a hospital. It can be understood how believing I am at work or in a hospital initiates an elopement behaviour – a need to leave the building for the simple reason "I don't belong here".

The resident's orientation is an important cue for members of the care team. If the resident has difficulty remembering where he is, he may also have difficulty relating to staff performing personal care. Imagine the conflict if a resident believes the unit on which he lives is his place of employment – no one at work attempts to drop my pants to take me to the bathroom. It is essential that on each contact staff reinforce to this resident where he is, who they are and what is about to be done.

67

Although such a basic approach may be thought common-place, it can be easily overlooked given the number of times it has to be done. Reminding all mentally impaired residents who you are and what you are doing each time you make contact becomes difficult considering the number of mentally impaired residents under your care, the number of times you may make contact with each in that day and the number of days you will be doing care.

It is more effective to identify to all team members those residents who become resistive or aggressive when not told where they are and who you are on every contact. Although that approach is encouraged with all residents, it is mandatory for those identified few. All staff (nursing, housekeeping, dietary, administrative, etc.) are expected to always reinforce with these specific residents where they are, who you are and what you are doing on every contact. By limiting the number of residents that need and can relate to this type of reinforcement, we have increased the chances that it will be consistently undertaken by all staff. If it is expected to be done with all residents, all of the time, the chances are great that the ones who need it will have it done, elevating their anxiety and causing frequent aggressive outbursts.

Impairment in recent memory is one factor contributing to the inability to remember where one is. Understanding what someone is talking about is another. As peculiar as it may sound, a mentally impaired resident "did not see himself come into the building". At the time of admission, the degree of anxiety experienced by this person probably resulted in his not seeing the building in which he was admitted. After living on the unit for a period of time, a degree of familiarity may have been achieved, decreasing his anxiety level. Once his anxiety has been lessened, he is more attentive to his surroundings, but all he can see are the interior walls of a building, some beds and furniture – easy to mistake that as home; or "nurses" – those in white uniforms – must be a hospital. The name of the facility means nothing if you cannot associate it with a building.

To associate the name to a building, the building must be seen. This can be established when residents are taken on walks outdoors. When outside, the resident's attention needs to be brought to the exterior of the building, at the same time a picture of the exterior of the building is shown to the resident and the name of the facility and its function is reinforced (Home for the Aged, Nursing Home, etc.). A similar picture, blown to a larger size is in the resident's lounge, with the name and function of the building in large print above it. To some residents this association may be of value in identifying their location.

It is important to reinforce that the severity of a resident's impairment becomes the key factor in determining the success of such cuing. Low functioning mentally impaired often cannot relate to such an abstract and complex mechanism.

Again staff become the main source of the information – where the person is, who they are and what they are about to do. Some residents will have no ability whatsoever to recall where they are. Anticipation and constant reinforcement becomes the only realistic approach.

c) Person

Some mentally impaired residents can remember faces and names, some can only remember faces, others can remember neither.

A daughter was introducing me to her mother. The mother suffered from Alzheimer's disease and had very poor recent memory retention. Once the introduction was made, the mother said to me "Who is that standing next to you?" It was the daughter. Mother was incapable of remembering the daughter by name or face. Once the daughter heard mother's question, she became incensed. "You know who I am mother. She always does this. She knows who I am when she wants." Wrong! Mother has lost the mental ability to identify most, if not all persons by name or by face. Yet the daughter would not accept her mother's limitation. I discovered that the daughter spent every visit attempting to have mother address her by name. You can imagine the result of such pressuring on the emotional state of both and how each visit ended.

This expectation that Alzheimer's victims have the ability to turn memory on and off is deleterious to effective care. It assumes that a person with a destructive brain disorder is able to be selective. That is impossible! Yet some will always argue – "My mother remembers my sister who rarely visits, but she never knows who I am. She is just trying to make me feel guilty for putting her in the nursing home." It is amazing how some insistently ignore the effects of the disease, insisting that cognitive functioning is still operable.

This often reinforces the need for staff to introduce themselves on each contact and explain what they are about to do. When working with a specific resident five days a week for two years, there develops a considerable degree of familiarity on the part of staff. We see that same resident each day, and easily can believe the resident has the same degree of familiarity. In actual fact to some residents, no matter the number of contacts made with staff, each time may be the first time.

Some mentally impaired are able to remember faces but not names. Certain staff will enter the room of a specific resident and get a very different response than others, such as a smile and a warm greeting. The same is true of family. When the daughter visits, the resident may greet her with a hug and a smile. Ask the resident who she is and she will probably respond "I don't know". The resident is responding to the familiarity of the face. There is some part of that face she can recall, telling her that she has seen this person before, but she cannot remember where or when. So she responds accordingly.

The ability to remember one face and forget another demonstrates well the spotty and random destruction occurring within the brain. There is no conscious, selectivity on the part of the Alzheimer's victim.

Assessment:

Does this person work here or live here?

Pointing to a resident and then to a staff member and asking the above question will provide considerable information. The ability to know whether the person you are pointing to lives or works here gives a possible indication of the resident's response to people approaching him. If incapable of differentiating between staff and other residents, there will be an obvious resistive behaviour to being taken to the washroom. Likewise, such a resident may mistakenly approach other residents for assistance in being toileted and the delay in finding the right person to take her may be the main cause for her incontinence.

d) Thing

The location of the damage in the brain dictates the information that is lost. A resident may have the ability to dress himself – no problem putting on his shirt, pants and socks, but when it comes to his sweater, he just stares at it. It is easy for some staff to interpret his actions subjectively, believing he wants attention or is just being difficult. In actual fact he may be demonstrating one very specific limitation – he has lost the ability to identify what a sweater is.

It seems that as parts of the brain are damaged, very selective pieces of information may be lost. In this instance he can recognize and manipulate most articles of clothing, but a sweater has now become a foreign object. The damage may be even more selective. He can identify a sweater but doesn't know what to do with it – where is the top, the bottom, the sides. The ability to manipulate a sweater is lost, all points of reference seem to be gone.

Assessment: What is this?

It is important to determine which objects in every day use the resident is capable of identifying. While interviewing or performing care, simply point to a common object and ask "What is this?" If he is repeatedly incapable of correctly identifying many objects, then it is important to know what this person can recognize and what he cannot. This information becomes essential for all staff in knowing what instructions must be given to him, what should be asked of him and what supports he will require.

An item as simple as a chair can create specific problems for some mentally impaired. A staff member pats the back of a chair and asks Mr. Jones to sit down, and he does. A short while later that same staff member says to Mr. Jones "Please go and sit in the chair." He doesn't respond. He doesn't know what a chair is, but when he sees one he knows what to do with it.

To associate a specific word (chair) to the appropriate object requires the person to first form a mental image of that object then compare that image to something found in the environment that is identical. That is simple enough to demonstrate:

I will provide the following word:

TREE

Now find one! In order to find a tree, you must compare the picture you created in your mind's eye with something identical in the environment. If you were unable to create an image of a tree in your mind, how would you find one?

For some mentally impaired, the information required to create the image is lost, making the words meaningless. Some residents who may not be able to identify an object by name, may still use it and respond appropriately if they see the same item (chair). If staff are not aware of this limitation with a specific resident, it could easily lead to labeling that person as attention seeking or resistive.

Without knowing what a resident can identify by word or by sight, it is impossible for staff to determine how to communicate effectively to any resident and be supportive of their limitations during care.

MEMORY

The inability of the mentally impaired to retain recent memory is the main premise for many limitations. In fact Alzheimer's Disease can be referred to as "Reversed Aging". As the disease progresses, more recent memory is lost. Initially the resident may be able to remember up to a month ago. As more and more of the brain is damaged, further memory is lost. At some point the person may be able to recall only specific events that happened years ago.

One of the challenges in working with the mentally impaired is to determine how much memory has been lost. Some are unable to remember much of the past 40 years, but can converse in depth about the most minute detail that occurred on a specific day in the 1940's. This contradiction in ability creates considerable confusion on the part of some family members – "How is it that Dad can remember little things that happened years ago, but can't remember that I visited yesterday?"

Probably the most basic way to imagine the progression of memory loss in association with the related brain damage is to compare the brain to an onion. Imagine the brain layered like an onion, where recent memory is in the outer layers and older memory closer to the core. As the brain is being destroyed take a layer away. This analogy serves two purposes. The first is to demonstrate the progression of memory loss as the disease worsens. The other is to display the permanency. Once a layer of an onion is removed, it cannot be replaced. It is gone. Likewise with the destructive nature of the disease, once memory is lost, it is lost and cannot be put back.

The ability to remember certain aspects of one's life and its past is totally dependent on the location and degree of destruction within the brain. Selective areas of the brain can be destroyed. Whatever information those cells retained will be lost. This emphasizes again the error in comparing one Alzheimer's victim to another. Staff who believe that both Alzheimer's victims in a semi-private room know who she is and what she is doing, because one has such an ability would have disastrous results.

Assessment:

How old are you?
What is your spouse's name?
How many children do you have?
What are their ages?
I will give you three words – house, orange and dog.
I would like you to remember them (in 5 minutes ask what those words were).
My name is _____ (in 5 minutes ask if he knows your name).

Each of these questions is an opportunity to determine the degree of memory loss experienced. The inability to recall the interviewer's name or three simple words is a good indication of the resident's difficulty with recent memory. This person would probably demonstrate a significant problem in following instructions, requiring staff to repeat to him what they want done rather than expecting him to remember the sequence in total.

The challenge is to know what the person can remember. One of the most effective assessment strategies of supportive therapy is to personify – "to get inside that person's head". Personification is an attempt to know what the person can remember in order to understand his behaviour and adjust interventions and approach appropriately.

Some may believe that such a feat is impossible or useless. On the contrary, personification is one of the key skills in achieving empathy, the ability to place ourselves inside the head of the person under our care. I do not know what it is like to have cancer, be dying or be severely depressed, but through increased contact with those in these states, the opportunity to intuitively understand that person's frame of reference increases. That understanding can be encountered when working with the mentally impaired elderly as well.

One Alzheimer's victim, when asked the year, would always place his answers around the "1950's". Staff and family found that he was continually obsessed about money, always telling staff he didn't have enough money, trying to pay staff as soon as they completed a task for him, never letting his wallet out of his sight, talking about going to the "poor house" and so on. To staff this behaviour had little meaning until they talked with the resident's daughter. From his daughter, staff learned that in the late 1950's this resident owned and operated his own business. Due to financial difficulty, his business went bankrupt. For a period he was unemployed. During that time he was constantly fearful of the family's financial survival. It is not always as obvious as in this case, but if you can identify where the resident is in time, you may understand the behaviours he is presenting.

One very important question that must be asked of family to assist in understanding where that mentally impaired resident may be locked in time is "What significant events stand out for you about your mom/dad's life?" Memory is selective. We do not remember every minute of our life. Instead we will remember things that have associated with them strong emotions, whether positive or negative.

To demonstrate, imagine the following:

> Go back in time/
> To the first day
> You brought home your first child/
> Remembering all of the things that happened on that day/

For most, such memories would elicit a smile. What happened the second day? Unless something unusual occurred, most would not be able to recall that day or the next. Often what we will remember are things that have attached to them strong emotions, either positive or negative. To prove that further, how often have you recalled an event you "screwed up" 10 or 15 years ago? For most, that event still stands out in our mind. Knowing that memory is strongly attached to emotions gives us a clue on working effectively with the mentally impaired. The more we know of that person's past, the more we may understand his present behaviour.

The mentally impaired are virtually in a time warp. They interpret events, people and situations based on their place in time. If a female Alzheimer's victim believed she was in her past, at a time when she had a child who was gravely ill, her behaviour would be obvious. Each time that memory was recalled, it would entice her to look or call for that baby even though now she is 80 years old and living in a long term care facility.

We have just demonstrated an important aspect of understanding certain behaviours of the mentally impaired – to the mentally impaired, their world is very real and they respond accordingly.

A gentleman (94 years old) and his wife (87) were living in a long term care facility. The husband was well, both physically and mentally, living on the independent wing of the facility. The wife suffered from Alzheimer's disease, was very impaired and lived on one of the nursing units. I was asked to counsel the husband who was having great difficulty with his relationship with his wife.

He stated "When I walk into me wife's room and she sees me, she tries to hit me, bite me and sometimes spit at me. When she sees my son, she calls him by my name. When she sees my daughter she calls her by her mother's name." The goal again in supportive therapy is to attempt to understand the world of the individual under your care – to personify. This method of getting inside that person's head allows one to speculate what that person sees and experiences. I asked the husband for a recent picture of his son. He showed me a picture of a 64 year old man that was the spitting image of his father. When I assessed the wife, her thought process was fragmented and disjointed, but everything she discussed placed her in her 50's.

Imagine her situation. She is sitting in her room. In her mind she is in her 50's, and in walks her 64 year old son. To her he looks just like her husband. In walks her 67 year old daughter, who possibly looks like her mother. She has it straight. She is in her 50's, her son is her husband, her daughter is her mother. Then in walks her 94 year old husband. Who does he look like? Like her husband only older. I was able to identify the resemblance of the son and father immediately by the photograph of the son. Who does he say he is? Her husband. Now she becomes confused. Her anxiety is elevated, she is out of control and becomes aggressive.

In talking with the husband, I encouraged him that when he visits his wife he cannot keep stressing that he is her husband.

To see if the visits could be less stressful, he should visit more as a friend. He made another choice. Not to visit at all. He could no longer tolerate the aggressive outbursts of his wife and believed that he was making her situation worse. His response "I have been married to that lady nearly 70 years. I can't treat her only as a friend. It is better not to visit." He defined well the dilemma and pressures experienced by family (discussed in chapter fourteen).

This can also work in the positive. On one unit, the majority of staff had difficult getting a mentally impaired lady to take a bath. When the case was reviewed it was found that one staff (Rose) had relative ease in completing the task. To this resident, Rose was a long lost friend. The resident would do anything for her. There was something about Rose, her hair style, colour, facial features or body shape that hooked into the resident's past memory. This resident is back at that time in her memory process and therefore was willing to allow Rose to perform any care.

This emphasizes a very significant point in the care routine of that unit. It was asked why this resident's bath day was restricted to Tuesday only? To have the routine so restrictive, required whoever was on duty that day to battle through the bath. Instead, this resident's bath should have been scheduled on "Rose's day", being completed only when that specific staff member was on duty, regardless of which day it was. This ensured that the care process was both supportive to the resident and the staff required to do the care. The team had to be flexible enough to adapt to the memory process that was occurring and utilize the resources they had available to them.

AFFECT

Affect refers to emotion. One of the most common emotional states of many mentally impaired is a flat affect – no or little emotional expression. This person seems to have few highs and few lows, rarely seen to be laughing or crying. He sits expressionless, whether alone or involved with others.

One daughter said to me "My father hates me!" I asked how she knew that. She responded "I placed my father in the home when he became too much to handle. Every time I visit, he refuses to smile no matter what I do." The problem isn't that he will not smile, but he cannot. For this individual, the area that controls emotional expression is severely damaged. The person with flat affect has lost the ability for spontaneous emotional expression. That means he cannot take what feelings he is having on the inside and express them non-verbally through a smile, facial expression, eye movements. Subjectifying this limitation can be deadly for family or staff.

This person's inability to express emotion must not be mistaken as apathy or an unwillingness to be involved. The centre for emotional control in the brain has been damaged, blocking the person's ability to express any emotional spontaneity. It is important for family to be made aware that dad's lack of expression is not an indication that he has no feeling for them, but only an indication that he is limited in his ability to express it.

In fact some staff will say "There is no use bringing him to any activities he never seems to enjoy them." The question must be asked "When he attends an activity does he participate or observe?" If the answer is "yes" to either, then keep taking him to the activity.

By the way, a person with a flat affect will rarely become aggressive. Not only may he be unable to express happy or pleasant emotions, but angry ones as well. There are limitations to this. Like everything else discussed, there is no such thing as black or white answers to such limitations. For some experiencing a flat affect, a response may be elicited at certain times. The person rarely smiles, but if you place your face right in front of his, smile or laugh in his direct view, he may respond with a smile in return. That smile will be quickly lost when you withdraw. Likewise, pull this person out of a chair or speak loudly and aggressive to him and you may get a brief aggressive response that is soon lost. This demonstrates that for some, if the stimulus is intense enough you may be able to elicit a response.

The other and more difficult emotional change that may occur with mental impairment is a volatile affect. This is the resident who is sitting quietly and for no apparent reason becomes aggressive. This aggression may last for 20 minutes or 20 seconds and for no apparent reason it stops. Emotional control in this state is restricted due to the specific damage within the brain. This can occur when cells within the area of the brain that controls emotional expression have been damaged, but not destroyed. When damaged, they alter their functioning ability.

This situation can be compared to a person who experiences epilepsy. This is not to say that the interaction is the same, but if you understand epilepsy, you will better understand what is happening to the Alzheimer's victim who is volatile. An epileptic usually experiences some alteration to specific brain tissue. Under the right circumstances, those altered cells within that area become excited, stimulating the brain and causing a convulsion or seizure. Similarly, if cells that control emotional expression within the brain of an Alzheimer's victim are damaged but not destroyed, these cells could fire off, stimulating the area of the brain that controls emotional expression, causing an aggressive outburst. The person can be said to virtually experience an "emotional seizure".

Determining the pattern of such outbursts is significant in dictating the approach to be taken by staff. At such points in time the individual must not be pushed to be involved in any activities, whether bathing, eating or dressing, etc. Instead, he should be placed in a safe environment, away from any stimulus until it runs it's course.

PERSISTENT STIMULI AND REPETITIVE BEHAVIOUR

We have all encountered the Alzheimer's victim who persists in tapping on the table or repeating the same words again and again – "1, 2, 3 . . . 1, 2, 3 . . . 1, 2, 3 . . ." or "Mother, mother, mother . . .". Unfortunately, some who do not understand the mentally impaired will say that this behaviour is intentional – a conscious attention seeking mechanism that the resident can turn on and off at will. Their proof is that the resident mainly demonstrates this behaviour when he is sitting quietly alone. He slows or stops the behaviour when you get him talking or doing something. They believe that when you give him the attention he wants he will stop, only to start again when you walk away. That assessment is completely wrong!

This process can be called the Persistent Stimuli Effect. It can occur in many parts of the brain causing repetitive and bizarre behaviour in emotional expression, motor movement or even tactile response. What may be occurring may be similar to the process causing volatile affect. An area of the brain is damaged but not destroyed. The cells in that damaged area have been altered. They are highly excitable and virtually always at an "on" position, firing off low voltage at regular or irregular intervals. When the cells in the affected area fire, they stimulate that part of the brain to respond. If located in the area of speech, the person will repeat the same word again and again. In contrast, when distracted by someone walking in, talking to him or having him do another task, another part of the brain is stimulated or excited. The intensity of the electrical activity of this area is greater than the area creating the repetitive speech. It has the power to override the affected area. Once the person leaves, that area of the brain shuts down, and the affected cells with the low random voltage controls the brain once more, starting the repetitive behaviour or speech again.

Whenever the person is sitting quietly, the damaged cells dominate the brain. The only time this person may be able to stop the behaviour is when he is completely asleep.

This behaviour is very individualized. For some Alzheimer's victims it begins later in the day. In the morning there is no repetitive speech. As the day progresses, it increases with intensity and frequency. The attributing factor may simply be the person's tiredness level. During the morning the person is well rested and able to use what remaining mental ability there is to concentrate on the movement, noise and stimuli around him. He is keeping his mind active. As long as it is active, the affected area is overridden and unable to stimulate the repetitive behaviour. As the day progresses, the resident becomes more tired and the affected area is able to dominate and the repetitive speech pattern will begin.

It becomes even more complicated. The person may become extremely sensitive to the stimuli around him, where the activity level influences his repetitive pattern. Staff have seen this. When the unit is noisy and there is considerable movement around this resident, the repetitive speech will be faster and louder. When the unit is quiet it is less frequent and lower in volume. The stimuli of a noisy environment is indiscriminate. There is no one sound to focus on. The entire brain is excited, exciting the affected area further, increasing the frequency and volume. On the contrary, when the unit is quiet, this person's brain is at rest and the repetitive pattern decreases.

This same repetitive pattern can occur with motor movement. This is the resident who continually taps on the top of a table or arm of a chair. Some staff will again believe it is intentional, attention seeking behaviour, where the resident can control his movement at will. Impossible! Instead, it is an unconscious, spontaneous, spastic movement. It can best be compared to a person suffering from Parkinson's disease. Again, I am not implying that the same process is occurring, but if you understand one you will more clearly understand the other. A person with Parkinson's will demonstrate the "pill rolling effect" of the fingers, constantly moving his thumbs against his finger tips. If you ask that person if he is aware of his movement he will probably respond "I have been doing it so long I am not conscious of it." If you ask him if he can stop. He will now take an unconscious act and make it conscious. Flexing the muscles in his hands and forearms, slowing or possibly stopping the movement. Once he removes his concentration, the movement re-occurs.

Ask an Alzheimer's victim who is tapping the table top if he is aware of what he is doing. If he can understand your question he will probably respond "No I'm not!" His movements are an unconscious and spontaneous spastic act. Ask him to stop the behaviour. Again if he can understand your request, he will take an unconscious act and make it conscious. He will flex the muscles in his arms, which will slow the movement or possibly even stop it. Once his concentration is removed, the tapping will begin again.

This persistent stimuli effect can occur with tactile sensation as well. Low functioning mentally impaired residents will often be seen scratching at a certain location on their body repeatedly, possibly to the point of drawing blood and ulcerating that area. This person may even comment "Bugs, take the bugs away." The resident is not hallucinating, but trying to interpret what is being experienced. What may be occurring is similar to what was described earlier. The area of the brain that controls tactile sensation of the forearm is damaged. The cells are being stimulated again and again, providing a brushing sensation to that area. The resident only experiences the feeling and associates it with "bugs" brushing her arm. In this instance it is obvious that this resident's finger nails must be short and clean. In some situations gloves may be merited to prevent serious injury.

In each of these situations there is little that can be done medically to stop the behaviour. Giving enough medication to stop the repetitive activity would result in sedating the resident to the point of being non-functional. That option is not in keeping with the mandate of providing quality of life. The only thing that staff can do is to learn to live with it. Each staff member must define her own tolerance level – how long she can work with this resident before her patience runs thin. Everyone has a different tolerance level with each behaviour. Some can last the shift without it bothering them, others only a few hours. Once that limit is reached, staff must have the freedom to say so and then assign the resident to someone else for the remaining time. For staff to lose their patience, is to lose control, which is a dangerous situation in any care setting.

Likewise, it must be determined how long the unit or other residents can tolerate the repetitive pattern. This resident may have two sitting areas, one in the lounge and one in his room. When the behaviour becomes disruptive to the others on the unit, the resident needs to be removed from the common lounge and placed in a comfortable location in his room until the unit calms down, then returned again to the lounge. Unfortunately, the only thing that will stop this behaviour is when that part of the brain is completely damaged. This is an indication that the disease process is worsening.

COGNITION

Cognition refers to problem solving ability. Those with difficulties in cognition have difficulty with sequential thought. To the mentally impaired with an impairment in cognition, each task has the potential of only becoming a series of problems. Whatever this individual is required to do presents itself into specific isolated components that must be resolved.

If you ask a resident "Please go to your room", the problems presented are immediate. Which door do you take? Once you decide on a specific door then it is not only which direction do you go – forward, left or right, but also where did you "come from". The mentally impaired who have difficulty with cognition or sequential thought will have problems keeping their thoughts in order. Hence, every task may present itself as a series of problems. Problem solving involves abstract thinking, a significant limitation to many of those who are mentally impaired.

In fact, limitations in problem solving ability can be so impaired in some that it even effects their wandering ability. When such an individual encounters an obstacle (a secured door or a wall), it creates a major problem that this person may be incapable of solving. On encountering an obstacle in the wandering path, this resident will still seem to attempt to go forward. Standing in front of the wall or door, the resident ends up walking in one place and will remain there until someone assists him to turn around and go in another direction. The problem encountered when standing in front of the door or wall is as follows – "I can't go forward, I don't remember where I have come from or where I am going. Now what do I do, where do I go and how do I get there, turn left, right. . . ?" It is not uncommon to find in some instances a unique relationship developing between this wanderer and another mentally impaired person on the unit who wanders. The pair seem to always walk together and when one hits the blockade and is stuck, the other, almost on cue, takes her by the shoulders, manually turns her and then they continue down the hall.

Limitations in cognition is significant in identifying the importance of clearly defined programming for the mentally impaired in two areas. First, it demonstrates the need for a clearly defined environment that communicates to the mentally impaired rather than requiring them to function by memory only. Secondly, it also shows the importance of communicating brief, one step instructions for even the simplest task. Each of these areas will be expanded further in subsequent chapters.

PROGRESSIVE APHASIA

This limitation varies from the ability to find specific words the individual wishes to express to the point where the person is non communicative. Often a person lacking the "right" word, will substitute it with another word or phrase that for them replaces it the best.

You have encountered in your care a resident who will say "change my pants". When you examine the gentleman you find he has not been incontinent. Over time you begin to learn that when he says "change my pants", he means take him to the washroom or you will have to change his pants. He has lost the ability to express what he is feeling, a need to go to the bathroom; or he has lost the ability to say or recall the word bathroom, so he replaces it with the next best thing – "change my pants" to communicate his needs.

Learning a person's vocabulary is important. A female resident who has lost the ability to say her husband's name or simply the word husband may develop her own specific way to communicate. She approaches you and says "Where is my brother?" Her brother may have just visited an hour before and when you tell her this her response will be "Not my brother, my brother". She now uses one word to convey two meanings.

Assessment: The Interview (discussed in chapter eleven)

The only way to determine a person's language is by conversing with him. When speaking with a mentally impaired individual it is important to consciously be aware of any patterns demonstrated. In this case identifying the number of times the person replaces or exchanges one word for another. This same approach is significant for any staff performing care. Identifying patterns where a resident constantly refers to "the rag" instead of the towel, or "the scoop" instead of a spoon, etc. is the key. You can imagine the elevation in anxiety experienced when the resident believes she is saying what she wants, but no one seems to understand her and she has no other way of expressing herself. Once staff are familiar with the person's language pattern, they have gained a significant asset in supporting this individual during any activity – understanding what she wants even though the words used have very different meanings.

PROGRESSIVE APRAXIA

This refers to the inability to perform purposeful activity. One of the effects of such a symptom seems to be the loss in hand–eye coordination and fine muscle movements. With this limitation the individual loses the ability to manipulate objects even though muscle control seems to be intact in every other way. Such a resident feeds himself by using his fingers rather than a fork or spoon regardless of the persistence of others. It becomes too difficult and frustrating to manipulate any utensils and easier just to pick up what you want to eat with your fingers.

A more serious consequence occurs as the disease progresses and the individual loses the ability to control the muscles to stand or walk safely. This is the resident who is wobbly, at a high risk of falling or the one who seems to have the greatest difficulty in rising from a chair.

DELUSIONS

Delusions are incorrect beliefs that remain despite all other evidence to the contrary. Such a resident identifies a staff member or another resident as a person who steals or hurts them or can't be trusted even though that person has done nothing to merit such an accusation.

Many of these beliefs may have a sound basis for the mentally impaired. This resident may be relating his accusation to the stimulus being received. He now sees in another person a characteristic, manner, expression or appearance that reminds him of someone in his past with whom he had a negative experience. That resident now associates that experience with this individual, and responds accordingly.

In fact, the anxiety state and memory loss of the mentally impaired may initiate from them a tendency to read things at face value. Seeing a specific nurse handling another resident leads to a belief that she may be hurting her and can't be trusted. Remember that to certain mentally impaired residents, this is not a long term care facility and we are not caregivers. Instead it may be work or a bus depot – "What is that young woman doing taking that old lady by the arm? She has no right doing that." An assessment of the situation based on the resident's perception.

The potential delusional effects encountered by the mentally impaired was demonstrated well on a unit I was assessing. The first person I encountered when I walked onto that unit was a lady in her seventies, who was very confused and disoriented. She took one look at me and yelled to everyone "Be careful of that Bugger. He's the one, he can't be trusted. Bugger, Bugger, Bugger, Bugger!" Something of my appearance clicked with this lady to initiate that response, for reasons known only to her. Possibly she has a mistrust of someone with a beard or I resemble someone she had a bad experience with in her past. In either situation there is little that could be done to correct her behaviour towards me. In this instant it was just a matter of time. The more I visited the unit, avoiding making direct contact with her, smiling if I met her in the hall (regardless of her salutation of "Bugger, Bugger ..."), the less she became threatened. There is no question that had I been required to care for her, there would have been tense moments. In this situation the best approach would be to have someone else complete her assessment. This will be discussed further under the chapter involving staff supports.

It is important to establish at this point that working with the mentally impaired can lead to some embarrassing moments or uncomfortable times if a staff member is not prepared for what she may encounter. Often this type of resident will say what first pops into his head regardless of how embarrassing or insensitive it may appear. Many mentally impaired lose the ability to inhibit thoughts or expressions as they did in the past.

In order to function in a socially acceptable manner, a person must be able to remember the rules of what is socially acceptable or not. With memory limited, rules are forgotten. So one blurts out whatever is on one's mind. This is complicated further by the person's egocentric–like response discussed earlier. In chapter one we demonstrated that the mentally impaired have a significant limitation in their awareness of the feelings of others. It is impossible to be sensitive to what can "hurt" or upset others when one is experiencing an intense anxiety state. In fact, the best philosophy in working with the mentally impaired is "to expect the unexpected". You will hear, see and experience almost anything with the variety of mentally impaired encountered. An important quality in the survival of any staff member is to just let it "roll off your back".

ILLUSIONS

There is considerable controversy whether Alzheimer's victim's hallucinate. It is my belief that it is not as common as once thought. To hallucinate is to see something that is not there. Instead it appears that the mentally impaired experience illusions rather than hallucinations.

An illusion is a misinterpretation of what is seen. One of the basic concepts discussed earlier was "if the stimulus is not intense enough, then it will be missed or misinterpreted". That seems to be the most significant effect in describing the behaviour of many mentally impaired residents. They misinterpret what they see, feel or hear. If what the person is experiencing is not intense enough he will relate to it based on what he believes it is.

Many examples demonstrate this well. The resident who bends down frequently to clean the dirt off the floor. Even though staff can see no dirt and attempt to correct her, she is adamant it is dirty. What this person may be seeing is the patterns in the tile or often the numbers of a shuffle board game painted on the hallway floor. These markings are not clear and to the resident they may look like smudge marks or dirt causing her to attempt to remove it.

One gentleman each evening at dusk would call the staff to look out his window at the kids playing in the yard. When staff looked out all they could see were small evergreen trees scattered throughout the yard. To this man, those tress appeared as small children playing in the yard.

Another lady insisted that her daughter was in the hallway, on the other side of a secured door. In fact what this resident heard was the voices of female staff walking down the hall and past the door. She interpreted these voices as her daughter talking to someone. This was perfectly logical given her frame of reference. Due to her memory impairment she believed that she was living at home with her daughter who was a young child. It made perfect sense that one of the female voices she heard on the other side of the door had to be her daughter's. A very accurate analysis given the cuing she experienced.

The challenge is understanding what it is that the mentally impaired see or hear and how they interpret it within their reality. The ability to personify – learning first where that person may be locked in time and then scanning the environment around him to identify what may be triggering off the associated behaviour. Once defined, then the ability to be supportive is increased allowing for appropriate interventions to be implemented specific to that person's needs.

HOARDING AND RUMMAGING

This refers to a resident's persistent gathering of belongings and objects. A number of factors can lead to this behaviour.

We have already identified the tendency of the mentally impaired to be constantly looking for something familiar in order to gain the security needed. As the resident walks around the unit, she discovers objects that are similar to the things she owns or once owned – a hair brush, matches, towels, etc., it is natural for her to believe these belong to her. So she gathers them up and places them in her room, if she can find it. Telling this person these are not hers often is fruitless and may even result in an agitated response. To her it is obvious those items are hers.

Another factor that can elicit rummaging behaviour is simply old behaviour. If the individual, all of her life, was a "neat freak" – having everything in it's place and a place for everything, then the behaviour to keep things in order may persist. As she walks about the unit, she finds things that she believes are out of place. It makes sense for her to put them where they belong. Depending on the degree of recent memory loss experienced, once she picks it up, she has forgotten what she was going to do with it and places it down in another location – false teeth in the toilet bowl.

SUSPICION

Remembering that many mentally impaired will interpret actions and stimuli at their face value and that interpretation is based on their existing mental frame of reference, it is understandable that suspicions exist.

Simple things like losing objects and believing you know where they are or should be or where you saw them last, makes you wonder who is playing games on you when you cannot find them in that location. Losing track of time and the loss of recent memory contributes to the fact that where you saw them last and where they actually were are not necessarily the same place. You saw them there months ago, but to you that was yesterday. The response "Who stole them?"

Actions of others become a significant stimulus to initiate suspicious behaviour. Hearing others talking but not being able to hear what they are saying becomes fertile ground to believe they are talking about you. Encountering another resident who is aggressive or loud and boisterous can be interpreted as a person who is out to get you.

Even the association with people and events you have experienced in the past that are now brought into memory influence your beliefs in what you now see. A female resident who is suspicious of male residents or staff being sexually aggressive toward her may be reliving a very bad experience in her past regarding a related incident. If she was sexually assaulted or abused when she was young, she may now be locked onto that memory, believing now that every man she sees is out to hurt her.

DECREASED ATTENTION SPAN

Depending on the severity of recent memory loss, concentration is easily impaired. Recent memory loss can be so intense that when an individual leaves her room planning to go to the dining room, she forgets where she is going once she walks through her bedroom door. Such an individual would have considerable difficulty performing any tasks that have multiple steps, following any instructions, or even maintaining a conversation.

To perform a task requires an individual to remember a sequence of events – what was just completed and what needs to be completed now. The person begins to eat, becomes distracted and then leaves the table, forgetting about the food that was left behind. Similarly, when asked to perform an activity, instructions are lost, concentrating on step one the person forgets step two and loses track of the entire process, until the sequence is easily abandoned. At that point it is easy to be distracted and wander away from the activity.

That explains why many mentally impaired residents have difficulty carrying on a conversation for any length of time. Conversation requires considerable concentration. In order to successfully maintain a conversation, the resident must be able to remember what was just said in order to determine a response. Poor recent memory easily knocks that sequence off balance. The person finds it difficult to keep track of the topic and rambles from one issue to another.

MIMICKING BEHAVIOUR

Some mentally impaired will wander as a result of mimicking behaviour. Wandering is a common and very complex symptom that will be discussed in detail in a following chapter.

Certain mentally impaired residents will mimic almost any behaviour – wandering, restlessness, agitation, etc. We established earlier that if the stimulus is not intense enough it will be missed or misinterpreted. For some mentally impaired the opposite is also true – if the stimulus is too intense they cannot help but respond.

IF THE STIMULUS IS TOO INTENSE,
SOME CANNOT HELP BUT RESPOND

Within minutes of staff sitting at a dining room table for a care conference, who is sitting around them? The stimulus is too intense. Residents wandering about see a group of people sitting at a table. The need to investigate in order to understand the environment elicits a response that might be compared to – "I wonder what they are doing? I will find out." Then that person sits with the group.

Even restless behaviour can be contagious. One female resident on a unit for the mentally impaired was a full time caregiver. Not a nurse or social worker, but throughout her life she would always search for those in need – disabled, mentally handicapped, financially impoverished – and help them, whether they wanted her help or not. Now she was on a unit with 30 mentally impaired older people. To her this must have seemed like "manna from heaven". At mealtime, like many caregivers, she would never think of sitting down and eating before all the rest at her table were settled and eating. Staff would place her plate in front of her, but she would stand up and go to the resident sitting next to her, saying "How are you dear? Look you have too much of this, let's give some to him and he has too much of this, let's give . . ." She would proceed to take food from one resident and give it to another. Eventually every resident at that table was into everyone else's food. They began mimicking her restless behaviour.

Some mentally impaired will mimic agitation. On another unit there was a female resident in her nineties that staff referred to as "the Screamer". Whenever she was placed at a table she would pound on it and yell at the top of her lungs "LUNCH, LUNCH, LUNCH, LUNCH, . . ." The effect her screaming and pounding had on other residents was to create a scenario that resembled a prison riot. Residents sitting in the dining room at her table who normally could concentrate on their meal and were fairly quiet, began screaming and hitting the top of the table, mimicking her behaviour.

SUMMARY

The symptoms of the mental impairment are many and complex. Each mentally impaired resident is different in the combination and severity of the symptoms experienced. Therefore there can be little universality in the approach and care concepts implemented. This individuality requires that programming be determined not by the person's diagnosis, but by his strengths and limitations. What is done to achieve quality of life for each resident is dictated by what he requires at any given time.

Before we can examine specific interventions required for effective caring for the mentally impaired elderly, it is important to relate these symptoms to the day–to–day encounters of the caregiver. It is one thing to talk about what the person can or cannot do, it is another to identify how his actions effect care and the ability of staff to be supportive.

Chapter Five

The Challenges in Care

What has been described to this point must be related to the day-to-day experiences of the caregiver. Understanding the sensitivity of the mentally impaired to their environment and the circumstances they encounter becomes the first step in being able to adjust one's approach and interventions to effectively provide this group with the most positive environment given their existing strengths and limitations.

FUNCTION/NOT FUNCTION

The most obvious trait of the mentally impaired is that even though they may function and behave in a certain manner at one time, their abilities and behaviour will be completely different at another. It seems that certain circumstances and specific times of the day can influence functioning ability – being able to function or not function given the right circumstances.

a) In Performing Tasks

Imagine:

> You are caring for a mentally impaired resident
> You sit her at her bedside/
> Give her a basin, a towel and a face cloth
> She washes her face and hands/
>
> It is Tuesday morning/
> You take that same resident for her weekly bath
> You place her in the tub
> Hand her the face cloth

She just stares at it/

There are many factors that come into play to possibly create this change in functioning ability (being able to wash one's face and hands in one location and not in another), they are:

1. Need to Adapt
With the mentally impaired elderly, any task that is changed slightly, makes it a new task. Adjusting to change requires a very complex, abstract cognitive process – effective problem solving ability must be employed in order to adapt. The "new" situation must be compared to the "old" one, identifying what part of it has changed, and then deciding what must be done now in place of the previous actions in order to be as successful.

To many mentally impaired residents this level of cognitive functioning is impossible. The slightest change in the environment or what is being asked may result in any task appearing to this resident as though it were new. The demand to adapt may mean a loss in the ability to successfully function.

This limitation can be encountered when a resident experiences a simple change in location or position – from sitting at the side of the bed with a face cloth and basin to sitting in a tub with just a face cloth. While in the tub how do you get the face cloth wet and where do you wring it out? Placing it in the water at your lap is much different from placing it in the water in a basin.

2. Moving From The Familiar to the Unfamiliar
We have established that changing a mentally impaired resident from the familiar to the unfamiliar increases anxiety. When anxiety increases mental functioning ability decreases. A task a resident may be able to perform in one setting may be lost in another, simply due to one's emotional state. Moving this resident from her room, where there is considerable familiarity, to the tub room that she encounters once a week will have that effect. Being in the tub room last week does not mean she remembers where she is now. She can easily be distracted by the noise, lighting, equipment, and staff movements of this new environment. Asking her to use the face cloth in this new environment causes considerable difficulty. She cannot concentrate on the task and is easily distracted by the new stimulus.

3. Bombarding

> What happens if a mentally impaired person is asked to do 10 things at once?

Usually that resident is unable to perform any of them successfully. Asking a resident to wash her face and hands at her bedside requires her to concentrate only on one task. Asking her to do the same task in the tub is very different. In the tub room she is exposed to a number of things all at once. To demonstrate the pressures, have that mentally impaired resident be you.

Imagine:

> I take you to the tub room/
> You are afraid I may leave you there alone
> Are you going to make it out to lunch/
> Are you in the same building/
> I undress you completely
> Get you in the tub
> Is the water too hot or too cold
> You have to wash your face
> Your arms
> Your neck
> Chest
> Torso
> Legs
> Feet
> Hair
> Get you out of the tub
> Get dried
> Dressed
> Leave/

All in 10 minutes!

Bombarding is asking an individual to perform multiple, separate tasks in a short duration. The usual consequence is the person is unable to perform any successfully.

Imagine what that mentally impaired resident goes through. Each task requires considerable thought and concentration. As the resident is working to complete one task, it becomes impossible to analyze quickly enough what has to be done to be prepared for the second one. Each bit of information and expectation only further complicates what has to be completed. This saturation of stimuli intensifies anxiety, limiting cognitive ability even further.

Staff who can relate to this change in functioning adjust their demands on the resident accordingly – assisting the resident where needed without criticism. Staff who view the change subjectively, usually believe that if this resident can perform in a certain manner in one location, then she should always be able to perform in the same manner regardless of place or time. Any alteration in performance is interpreted as a conscious decision by the resident to be resistive or attention seeking. Such a belief results in pressuring the resident to perform to the same level of competence as she did in her room – while the resident is sitting in the tub staring at the face cloth, this staff member would probably encourage her by saying "Come on Mrs. Smith. You can wash your face and hands in your room. You can wash your face and hands here." I truly hope that staff member has another uniform, for she may well be wearing that face cloth.

There is little difference between this scenario and the one identified in chapter two. In chapter two I had right sided paralysis, with a dead right hand. With that physical limitation, you would not consider pressuring me to "pick up my fork with my right hand". With this mentally impaired resident there is no difference in functioning abilities. Given the effects described above, she has been placed in a situation that is beyond her ability to cope. Any pressure to wash her face and hands on her own while in the tub will only result in increasing her frustration and anxiety level, leading to an aggressive response – the face cloth will go flying in retaliation.

It is not suggested that we take over every task for each mentally impaired resident who shows difficulty in functioning. Rather, this emphasizes that a universal approach in dealing with this clientele is not effective.

Certain impaired residents will only perform a task with strong encouragement. To constantly "take over" or rescue such an individual defeats the goal of Supportive Therapy – identifying the person's strengths and maintaining them. The main focus in approach is flexibility. Success in working with any resident is based on knowing that resident's abilities and limitations. That requires time and successful sharing among staff to ensure a consistent approach and realistic goals.

Those who have worked with the mentally impaired for any length of time (either staff or family) have discovered the best approach is one of trial and error. This is not a haphazard approach in dealing with the mentally impaired. It is a successful assessment strategy to determine the most appropriate programming. The process of using trial and error involves attempting something, observing the person's response and assisting when it becomes obvious the person's anxiety level is increasing. It is essential then that all staff involved in the care of this resident maintain the approach or programming that is discovered to be effective.

b) **During a 24 hour Period**

This Function/Not Function response can be further demonstrated when examining the potential changes a mentally impaired resident can encounter in a 24 hour day. Some residents seem to present three different "personalities" and functioning levels over three shifts.

How many times have you heard staff on the afternoon or nights shift say to day staff "I don't care what you say she does on days, she is not like that on our shift!"

The multiple changes experienced by a mentally impaired resident between day and afternoon shift become significant factors in dictating the behaviours he will exhibit. Let us examine the changes that can occur from the day shift to the evening shift to the night shift.

Day Shift to Evening Shift

1. Change in Staff Numbers
Usually on the day shift there are more staff on duty than during the afternoon shift. There are more nursing staff, plus housekeeping, recreation, dietary, volunteers and management staff coming and going. On the afternoon shift, probably only nursing staff are on duty at a reduced number compared to the day shift. The higher ratio of staff to residents on the day shift increases the frequency of staff/resident contact. Such contact increases the opportunity for a resident to be more oriented to his

surroundings, allowing him to respond more appropriately to what is requested of him. Conversely, a resident may be left alone for longer periods during the afternoon shift, increasing his disorientation, making him less cooperative.

A housekeeper is in the resident's bedroom every morning at 1000 hours cleaning. During that time in the room she converses with the resident. At 1015 hours the nurse enters the room to take the resident to the bathroom. The earlier contact with the housekeeper increases the possibility that the resident will maintain a better awareness of those around him and be able to respond more appropriately to the nurse when asked to move from one location to another.

On the afternoon shift the situation changes. A resident may have contact with a staff member at 1730 hours and not again until 1900 hours or later. During that period alone, the resident's orientation to his surroundings will probably decrease (past orientation discussed later – the longer you leave a mentally impaired individual alone, the more disoriented he will become). When staff attempt to take him to the washroom at 1900 hours, he may become less cooperative, not knowing immediately where he is and who this person may be. A significant change in functioning is shown over a 12 hour period.

2. Change in Staff Approach

If on the day shift (or any other shift), staff are positive in their approach – giving the resident time to perform tasks, adjusting tasks as needed, being supportive and flexible in that person's routine – the resident's anxiety will be low, allowing the resident to perform at his maximum level. If during the next shift the staff on duty is more structured and task oriented – performing care in a hurried, somewhat forceful manner – anxiety will be increased. This change in approach will result in a resident no longer being able to successfully perform tasks completed easily on the previous shift.

This can be better demonstrated by the following: If staff on a unit can know who was working the previous shift without looking at the time sheet, but only by the amount of agitation and wandering of many of the mentally impaired on that unit, then you have seen the effect one staff member can have on the functioning level of the mentally impaired.

3. Change in Energy

I want you to imagine what it would be like to do a mentally taxing task for 12 hours straight without a break.

How would you be by the 12th hour?

Imagine what it is like for a mentally impaired resident on a unit from 0700 to 1900 hours. Every task, stimulus, noise, every person has to be continually analyzed. By the 12th hour she would be exhausted. Tasks easily performed earlier in the day, become more and more difficult as her energy is depleted. As she becomes tired, her tolerance level deteriorates, decreasing her ability to concentrate and perform the task effectively.

4. Change in Lighting

During the day, lighting is both direct and indirect – fluorescent lights above and daylight through the windows. Both sources of light make objects clearly visible.

Many mentally impaired residents develop "anchors" in the environment – using a specific object in a room to help identify their location, rather than trying to remember the room itself. Probably the best anchor utilized by many mentally impaired residents is a comforter or personal bedspread on their bed. As long as the resident can see his bedspread, he knows it is his room. To demonstrate how significant the bedspread is, just remove it from that resident's bed and place it on someone else's. Now that becomes that person's room. The room is found by locating the anchor or object.

Imagine:

I am a mentally impaired resident
Easily disoriented/
To locate where I eat
I wander
Until I find "my table"/
A long rectangular table in a corner
My chair where I normally sit is at the end/
At breakfast and lunch
I have no trouble finding "my table"/
I walk directly into the dining room unassisted/

At supper it is different/
I wander the halls
Requiring the staff to take me to the dining room for my
    meal/

During the day, the amount of light available makes "my table" clearly visible. During the evening the light changes. With the sun setting, the main source of light in the dining room is from the ceiling only. If that lighting is poor, it creates shadows. Shadows are an obscure stimuli (if the stimulus is not intense enough it will be missed or misinterpreted). The table now has a shadow along one side that makes it appear more square in shape than rectangular. As a result, I find the dining room on my own for breakfast and lunch, but at supper I wander aimlessly about the unit. At supper, I can't see "my table". The distortion created by the shadow makes it look different.

This effect created by a change in lighting can aptly be called the "sundown syndrome". Shadows will distort any environment. To have a room look one way during the day when lighting is intense and have every object cast a shadow during the evening will intensify one's confusion and disorientation.

The combined effects of all of these changes – changes in staff numbers, staff approach, energy and lighting – may have a significant effect on a resident's functioning level from day shift to afternoons.

You bring me my breakfast tray
I feed myself/
You bring me my lunch tray
I feed myself/
You bring me my supper tray
I stare at it/

Those who understand the mentally impaired and how they are affected by different events, will assist the resident during supper, realizing his needs change at certain times of the day. Staff who lack this sensitivity may view the resident's inability to feed himself supper only as a conscious decision to be difficult or gain attention. Such a staff member may respond to this resident at supper in the following way: "If you can feed yourself breakfast and lunch, then you can feed yourself supper.

Now pick up your spoon and get eating!" Such pressuring only results in the resident sending the tray flying off the table.

Some staff working the evening shift may even suggest another reason for this resident's resistance – "You know why he is not eating supper. We have less staff than day shift and he is attention seeking." There can be nothing more further from the truth.

Evening Shift to Night Shift

A resident wakes at 2 a.m., what does she experience?

1. Staff Change – This is the most devious staff change of them all. When she went to bed at 2100 hours, you were on duty. When she wakes at 0200 hours, I am on duty. Is this the same place? She didn't see the staff change. Her inability to relate to what happened causes further disorientation, increasing her anxiety level.

2. Total Darkness – We have already established that many mentally impaired identify anchors in their environment – one cue that will provide the needed information to tell them where they are. Darkness eliminates all cuing. When a resident awakes during the night, all she sees is darkness. It is easy to understand her disorientation.

3. False Cuing – During the night there are a number of cues that may be difficult for a mentally impaired resident to decipher. Waking at two in the morning and believing one is at home does not explain: why this peculiar shirt won't let me sit up in bed (restraint vest); why there are bars on the sides of the bed that won't let me get out of bed (bed side rails); who that person is in the next bed (roommate); and who is walking in with a flashlight (staff making rounds). The inability to clearly define these cues results in considerable fear over what one is experiencing.

4. Loud Silence –

> Tonight you are home alone
> The house is empty/
> You go to sleep/

At 3 a.m. you are awakened
By a sound you have never heard before/
Go back to sleep/

During the day and evening shift, background noise on the unit muffles anyone calling out from their room. During the night shift it is different. As a mentally impaired resident, I awaken at two in the morning easily believing in the dark that I am home. Suddenly in the silence I hear from the next room another mentally impaired resident responding to being changed – "LEAVE ME ALONE. HELP THEY ARE TRYING TO KILL ME!" – you expect me to go back to sleep?

5. External Factors – If an individual is on a sleeping medication, that medication has it's greatest impact during the early hours of the morning, greatly affecting their cognitive functioning ability. Also there is a chance that the resident will wake from a dream or a nightmare, not knowing what is real or imagined, an experience we have all encountered.

Mentally impaired residents who wake early in the morning experience considerable anxiety and intensified disorientation. Staff who relate well to this clientele know the best approach to employ – simply allow the resident to get up, take him to the lounge, give him a cup of tea and toast and talk to him for awhile. By this simple intervention, the resident is provided a degree of security, allowing him to become more oriented to his surroundings and to the people around him. After a few moments of personal contact the chances are the resident will return to bed and sleep the rest of the night.

Staff who are task oriented take a different approach. They dictate the "rules" (legitimate or not) that residents are to stay in bed and sleep until 6 a.m. So these staff struggle with this resident to keep him in bed and have him "go back to sleep". This only causes the resident to become agitated, further restricting his ability to sleep. The consequences of these actions does not end at the night shift. This resident's agitation will probably spill over to the day shift and possibly even the next evening shift resulting in all staff having difficulty performing care.

What is the difference – fighting with a mentally impaired resident to keep him in bed and to sleep; or allowing the resident to get up, get dressed, wander a bit and finally sit in a lounge chair and sleep till six. The most successful tactic in approaching the mentally impaired is flexibility. If you expect "normal" behaviour of this resident, you are expecting too much. There is no schedule the mentally impaired can maintain other than their own.

The difficulty staff encounter is when one staff member fires off a resident's panic level, creating an agitated or wandering response, then all staff are required to deal with the consequences. The lack of sensitivity to a resident's inability to function at certain times of the day given the reasons explained above will have detrimental results. The resultant aggression or panic state caused by the pressure to perform can last for hours. This impedes the ability of all staff to be effective in subsequent tasks or activities. Pressuring a mentally impaired resident to wash her face and hands in the tub when she is not able to function could effect her ability and performance at the morning's activity program, lunch, afternoon activity, supper and beyond.

LOOKS WELL, ACTS INAPPROPRIATE

Frustrations are frequently experienced by staff working with a mixed resident assignment on a unit where the resident population is integrated – cognitively well/physically disabled with the mentally impaired.

Imagine:

> You have an assignment of 10 residents
> Six are cognitively well, four mentally impaired/
> You walk into the room of your first cognitively well
> > resident
> Your expectations of this person's performance are high/
> She knows right from wrong
> She can problem solve
> When you give her specific instructions
>
> She can clarify them if she does not understand/
> If she needs anything, she will ask/
> You walk into the room of your next resident,
> Another who is cognitively well/

Again your expectations of her performance are high/

You enter the room of your seventh resident
This person is mentally impaired/
When you pull back the covers in his bed
You find that he is covered in his own feces/
With his hands smearing it about/

The automatic response by some staff may be "Mr. Jones get your hands out of there. How many times have you been told?" It becomes difficult to maintain one's objectivity under such circumstances. This scenario needs to be examined from both points of view, first the resident's and then the staff's.

Are the mentally impaired aware of being incontinent of urine or involuntary of stool?

Some may not, but a majority appear to be. Depending on the person's cognitive functioning level, if a mentally impaired resident is left sitting with her clothing wet for any length of time, she will usually become restless, at times attempting to remove the soiled clothing herself. When a mentally impaired resident is asked if the puddle or feces on the floor is from him, his response may be "not mine", even though it is obvious where it originated from. This is not to say the mentally impaired are aware of what they have done, but possibly more aware of there being a problem causing them to feel uncomfortable. Toilet training is the first thing we learn in our maturing years and the last sensation for many to lose. This may be the cause of many mentally impaired residents becoming embarrassed by what has happened and result in their unwillingness to admit to their incontinence.

If early in the morning a mentally impaired resident is lying in bed with the side rails up and he needs to go to the bathroom, what does he do? He hasn't the cognitive ability to use the call bell if there is one in reach. He wouldn't know that if he pushed the button a nurse would come and let him up. All he knows is he has to go. So he goes.

What may contribute further to the "smearing" of feces in the bed may be simple, most of our residents have been caregivers all of their lives, not care receivers. The majority have had a lifestyle which dictated that when they encountered a "mess" they would clean it up. Now in his bed is a "mess". He either hides it in his water jug so no one will know what he did (result of his embarrassment) or cleans it up (result of old behaviour). Being mentally impaired, the more he attempts to clean the "mess", the worse it becomes. The point being emphasized is the person is attempting to function at his maximum cognitive ability.

A staff member walks into the room and sees him smearing the feces about. It is easy to believe that he is "playing with it", not knowing he is trying to help. Some staff are able to maintain their composure and be objective about the situation, seeing it through the resident's perspective. Many of us have difficulty maintaining that degree of objectivity during every problem. Instead we find ourselves pressuring the resident to function as a "normal" person would, expecting him to know that what he is doing is "wrong", an expectation that is beyond his ability.

Staff on an integrated unit cannot be blamed for losing their objectivity. It is difficult to always remember that the person in front of you is mentally impaired when most of the morning you have been working with six cognitively well, physically disabled residents. Leaving the last cognitively well resident, one's expectations of that person's functioning was high – the person was able to understand what was expected of her, what was right and wrong. Walking into the room of your first mentally impaired resident is not enough to sufficiently change your perspective. You may have lowered your expectations, but not sufficiently enough to meet this person's cognitive functioning level. The problem is a simple one – take the feces off this resident and he looks just like all other residents. In other words, he looks normal but is acting inappropriately. It is difficult to adjust one's approach and expectations when you cannot see the limitations in order to judge the direction of care.

The frustrations experienced with a mixed resident assignment (cognitively well/physically disabled, and mentally impaired) is that staff in seconds must completely adjust their approach and expectations. Not an easy task for even the most skilled of staff. It is so easy to say something to a mentally impaired resident in such a setting, then turn and ask yourself why you said it. You become aware afterwards that he may not understand what you are talking about.

This scenario, which is so frequently encountered on an integrated unit, can be compared to taking a medical unit and psychiatric unit of an acute care hospital and intermixing them. This would result in staff caring for two patients in a semi-private bedroom, where one patient in the first bed is admitted for a cholecystectomy (removal of her gallbladder) and the other patient in that room is a full blown psychotic schizophrenic (severe mental disorder, that can present very bizarre behaviour) in an acute state. Would that staff member have difficulty performing care? Absolutely. So why is it that we should expect so much more from those who work in long term care. We have two specialties in long term care, caring for the cognitively well, physically disabled and caring for the mentally impaired elderly. The concepts of each is different than the other. Yet on an integrated unit there seems to be little sensitivity to the pressures it creates for staff. Perhaps we should examine levels of care assignments in general in our facilities before expecting too much from the caregivers themselves.

REACTIVE

What is frustrating in working with the mentally impaired is that we do not know what they see, hear or feel. How many times have you had an 80 year old mentally impaired resident come to you and say, "Have you seen my mother? I just saw her going down the hall!" No matter how often you tell her, "your mother died 30 years ago", she insists she just saw her.

We keep returning to that overriding emotion experienced by the mentally impaired – anxiety. Being in a world you do not understand, you invest energy to make sense of what is around you.

Whenever I encounter a resident who frequently sees her mother on the unit, I ask the person's family to sit with me in the lounge to identify any resident or staff coming and going that looks like their grandmother, their mother's mother. They are encouraged not to look at the fine facial features, but at build, hair style, etc. – the more global cues. Invariably we will find someone who looks like that resident's mother.

The resident is locked into past memories, at a time when her mother was alive and part of her life. When she sees someone walk by who has similar features to her mother (same body build, hair style, etc.) it is easy to believe that was her. The resident is reactive, responding to things as she sees, hears and feels them.

The world of the mentally impaired is very real. They will interpret what they see, feel and hear based on how it fits into their reality. There are many examples:

A chair leg that squeals as it is dragged across the floor may initiate a resident who has lived with a cat all of her life to respond "those boys are hurting the cat again".

Hearing her daughter out in the hall, when she really hears staff talking as they walk past the door.

Looking for the "baby" when she in actual fact is hearing another resident crying out in another room down the hall.

Seeing someone that resembles a person in their past and calling that person by that long forgotten name.

Our frustration as caregivers results from our inability to see the world as the resident sees it, making it difficult at times to be supportive when we don't know what we are to be supportive of. This only emphasizes the continual need to personify. To get inside that person's head. To always attempt to see the world as the mentally impaired may see it in order to understand their behaviour. Effective personification is the result of repeated exposure to that specific individual; determining patterns of behaviour to be able to identify what that person may be encountering; knowing this person's history or past; and having effective assessments tools at one's disposal.

PREMORBID PERSONALITY

This is an area that is often overlooked when discussing the mentally impaired. Many will talk about the personality changes experienced by the disease, but few talk about a continuation of the person's personality even though they have the disease. Premorbid personality means that the personality characteristics the person had before the disease may remain but are now exaggerated.

Imagine:

> My entire life
> My normal tone & manner of speaking
> Is loud & aggressive/
> In a conflict situation
> I only get louder, more aggressive
> And interject a few four letter words to emphasize my
>   point/
>
> I am now 78
> I still have the same boisterous manner/
> My wife who has been married to me for over 50 years/
> Has learned to cope with my volume and behaviour
> By going "deaf"
> Not listening to the tone or the words used/
>
> I am now 80 years old
> Mentally impaired
> A resident on your unit/
> Being under considerable stress and conflict/
> How do I talk to everyone around me?

The way I talk to everyone on the unit, especially those who perform my care, is loud and aggressive, with a flavouring of foul language. Change me! You will never change me! Now that I am mentally impaired, I may hold onto the things that are familiar more than ever before. I may cope with my situation in the same manner as I always have – loud and aggressive with some foul language to accentuate my point. The only difference now is that my cognitive impairment causes my behaviour to be more extreme than it was in my past. I am less able to restrain my actions and language.

In the past, prior to my impairment, my boisterous nature was still controlled somewhat by my sensitivity to the response of others. I would notice if I had gone too far by their reactions and tone down accordingly. Now that I am mentally impaired, that sensitivity is lost. I can no longer read in others how my behaviour and language has effected them – their facial expressions or actions no longer show me they are hurt or offended. Words in the past I would never say in mixed company, spill out now no matter who is around. The "taboos" have been forgotten.

The frustration with this resident occurs in the varied responses by staff to this behaviour. Some staff have no problem performing the necessary care with this type of resident, while others are constantly intimidated or at logger heads with him.

The staff who handle this situation well probably respond to his loud and boisterous manner in the same way as his wife during their 50 years of marriage – they will go "deaf" to his onslaught. These staff will listen to what he is saying, but ignore the manner in which it is said. Even at a team conference these staff will state – "Oh Len is no problem, he's just loud. You can do anything you want to him. He won't hurt you."

Staff who cannot "tune out", personalize each encounter, believing he "should" be able to control himself and understand that he is upsetting everyone by his language. The belief that his behaviour is within his control results in their attempting to subdue him, to make him more cooperative. Unfortunately their pressuring him to change has an opposite effect – it increases his anxiety, causing even more agitated behaviour. Some staff forget that even if he did quiet down when asked to, in no time he will forget what was asked and return to "his normal behaviour" within minutes.

This is not to suggest that limits should not be placed on a resident's behaviour. This person is living in a communal environment where the rights and safety of others must be maintained. What is being questioned is the manner in which these limits are imposed. Staff who can relate to such a resident, will take the first barrage of insults by ignoring it. By being supportive, they can usually calm him down to the point where he will speak more softly and complete the task asked of him.

Other staff by their approach are only successful in intensifying his behaviour, which may result in their requesting a more drastic option to be taken – sedate him to quiet him down.

The staff who work well with this resident are confused about the problem. They may return after a few days off, to find him sedated to control his "behavioural problem". They cannot understand why this resident is medicated and find the drug not only quiets him down, but decreases his ability to function at all other activities as well.

The interventions taken for a physically violent resident are a different matter (discussed in chapter ten). In this scenario, we are dealing with "old behaviour" that will be impossible to change given the circumstances encountered. To establish an effective supportive environment for this resident, staff who are successful in tuning out the loud, boisterous manner must share their skills with those who are not. In some settings that openness is not accepted. Certain staff who are not willing to learn from their peers may respond "I have worked with these residents as long as you. I don't need you to tell me what to do." Unfortunately such an attitude only limits the effectiveness of the team.

A similar conflict arises amongst staff with a resident who demonstrates another extreme in behaviour – the dependent resident.

> My wife and I have been married 50 years/
> In our marriage
> She was highly dependent on me for emotional support/
> Whenever a problem placed her under stress
> She would virtually cling to me until the problem was
>   resolved/
> Once I helped her resolve it, she would be fine/
>
> She is now 78 years old
> Mentally impaired
> And living on your unit/
> Experiencing considerable stress/
> How would she respond to it?

The stress and anxiety of living on the unit will initiate the same behaviour she demonstrated throughout her life – the need to cling. Living in a long term care facility, she will most likely cling to those who are closest to her – staff. Some staff have little difficulty with this behaviour, while others will find it an annoying pattern that needs to be broken.

Staff who have the fewest problems with this resident are those who find time to be with this resident beyond the needs of direct care. Throughout the shift, these staff will make a conscious effort to spend a few extra moments with her – "Mary, I'm just going to sort the laundry. Why don't you come with me" or "Mary I'm just doing some charting. Why don't you sit with me?"

Staff who cannot relate to this clientele will employ a different approach – "Mary, I don't want you following me around. You need to stay in the lounge." For every four hours this lady is not allowed to cling, how is she? What will she be like in 24 hours? After 24 hours of not being able to maintain her normal manner of coping with the stress, she will probably demonstrate some very bizarre behaviour due to the prolonged and intensified anxiety experienced.

Those staff who believe they can change this woman's behaviour will experience the greatest difficulty. Even if she were able to respond to their frequent requests for her not to cling, it would take only a few moments for her to forget what was asked and return to her normal pattern.

The conflict between these two groups of staff is even more frustrating than the resident's need to cling. Staff who cannot relate to this resident will express to those who can "Why are you babying her, spoiling her? She shouldn't be allowed to cling." An unjust criticism! What staff are doing is being supportive – maintaining for this resident an environment that will help her cope given the limitations she is presently experiencing.

SUMMARY

I am always amazed when I hear those who do not clearly understand the mentally impaired elderly state that caring for such an individual is custodial, with few rewards. Those that know this clientele understand the disease and the limitation in affecting its course, but know well the challenges and rewards. There is much that can be done to enhance this person's quality of life. Some look for sophisticated, highly technical interventions. Those exist, but we have demonstrated here that some of the more basic and straightforward approaches will have the greatest impact on determining the effectiveness for any caregiver in providing quality care.

There is one more area that must be expanded as we delve into the world of the mentally impaired – behaviour and emotions. We have established the foundation to understanding many of the perceptions of this clientele. Now we will attempt to move closer to understanding how they respond to what they see, hear and feel.

Chapter Six

Understanding Emotions and Behaviour

Anger, frustration, anxiety, depression, sensitivity, elation, excitement, exhilaration, frivolity, all are major components of the human psyche. Each in varying degrees will influence a person's perception, reaction, ability and state of mind.

There is little we know about the link of cognitive ability and emotions. They are not separate entities, but intertwined to effect each other equally. To believe a person in a level two state of functioning cannot experience a variety and range of emotional responses because of memory loss is too simplistic.

The mentally impaired respond to the world around them as <u>they</u> perceive it. Their ability to appropriately interpret cues and information may be limited, but the range of emotions available to them is still present. In fact, even though a person may have a flat affect, unable to express emotions, it does not mean that emotions are not felt. There is no question that as the disease progresses some emotions may be lost, some may become distorted and exaggerated, some over powering and ever present.

The challenge to the caregiver is to understand the impact of emotions in association with cognitive dysfunctioning. The mentally impaired respond in a personalized, reactionary manner – identifying a few bits of information from a given situation, interpreting it within their mental time frame and limited mental abilities, and then reacting in the manner available to them. The more we can understand their perceptions, the more effective our interventions and supports.

DEPRESSION

Depression is a debilitating disorder. If not recognized it can even incapacitate the ability of a cognitively well individual and decrease his effectiveness. The following is an attempt to understand depression as it would be experienced by anyone, depression as it may be experienced by the mentally impaired, and the importance of recognizing and dealing with it.

All residents of a long term care facility are potential candidates for depression given the losses they encountered that lead to admission. The natural response to any loss is to grieve. Depression is a major component of the grieving process.

In fact, depression in the frail elderly is the most common mental disorder (see text Working with the Frail Elderly, by Len Fabiano). In the cognitively well elderly it has the potential of mimicking the symptoms associated with Alzheimer disease. If overlooked and untreated it can result in significant confusion and disorientation.

The common symptoms characteristic of depression are also very evident in Alzheimer's victims:

Loss of appetite
Loss of weight
Decrease of energy causing lethargy
Constipation
Anxiety
Withdrawal
Retardation of thought and action
Feelings of worthlessness
Apathy to environment and activities of daily living
And *Confusion*

This is not to imply that all of these symptoms in an Alzheimer's victim are due to depression, but to demonstrate that depression experienced by an Alzheimer's victim will only complicate their situation further, decreasing mental functioning.

Probably the best way to define depression is by using the two words – Helpless and Hopeless.

Helpless – A feeling that there is no way of getting out of the "hole" I am in.
Hopeless – A feeling that there is no one who can get me out either.

One of the frequent characteristics of anyone who is depressed is the continual reference to the past – what can be termed "past orientation". This past orientation has a significant influence on a person's perception and cognitive state and is more than simply reminiscing.

The frequent discussion or desire of a depressed individual for the "good old days" is a wish to have one's life as it was before the loss occurred. They turn to a time when things were like they used to be, a time of familiarity, a time of control. The future to a person who is depressed shows little hope. The helplessness/hopeless feelings associated with depression creates a belief that nothing will brighten tomorrow. As a result, there is little sense investing any energy to change today. At this point in the grieving process, all that remains in the present is the painful thought and emptiness of what has been lost. On the other hand, the past is intact. It represents how things used to be. The times of accomplishments, positive emotions, memories and worth. A haven from the emotional pain and turmoil of what exists in the here and now that cannot be changed and from what is feared of the future that cannot be predicted or controlled.

The mentally impaired are not void of such emotions. In fact the opposite may be more accurate. Their emotional sensitivity to the circumstances they encounter may be even more intense than those experienced by the cognitively well. The mentally impaired may not know exactly what they have lost, but there is generally this constant perception that something is missing. The feelings of helpless/hopelessness would be the exact feelings encountered by many in such a cognitive state – a feeling that no matter what I do I cannot make sense of the world I am in and no matter what you do, you cannot make sense of it for me either.

To the mentally impaired the past is alive and real. It becomes "their" present and is easily accessed into existing memory. The present as we know it or recent events as we see them are cloudy and difficult to place into focus due to the effects of recent memory loss. Each reference to the present to the Alzheimer's victim has associated with it significant stress, where the information is generally unclear and hard to assimilate, creating the feelings of helplessness and hopelessness. A significant loss of control.

We have now linked this past orientation behaviour of the mentally impaired not only to organic changes within the brain, but to the feelings linked to depression. The feelings of loss, of being removed from the known, of being detached from the familiar, an emptiness.

This past orientation is not a conscious act. It is simply a response to the individual's existing state of mind and emotions. Recalling the past can achieve for the depressed mentally impaired four very necessary effects:

1. A Sense of Value
2. Eliciting Lost Emotions
3. Occupying Time
4. Providing Familiarity

1. A Sense of Value

I am 78 years old
Mentally impaired in a long term care facility/
What exists now is a mere shell of who I was/
In the present I have little worth
My importance, my contributions are all in the past/
My value is in my past/

I can go into my past at any time/
I can relive any accomplishment I can remember
By so doing I can re-create for myself a twinge of that
    value I once had/

A need for value or a sense of worth is not lost because of mental impairment. How often do we still find our mentally impaired residents attempting to be active, doing, participating. Often their behaviour shows a link to a past activity, constantly cleaning, folding, hand gestures simulating sewing, etc. These gestures strongly indicate a need for worth or value, a life long need that has been ingrained in many and now becomes only a continuation of the past.

2. Eliciting Lost Emotions

A significant factor contributing to past orientation involves feelings. The chronic feeling of the mentally impaired is anxiety. The stress created by this state can only be endured for a limited period of time. The inability to escape the situation physically provides only one other option – to escape mentally.

113

Even if the pace in the environment slows, it may still be too fast for some mentally impaired. For a person experiencing memory loss, every bit of information must be constantly analyzed – every noise, every face, every stimulus – in order to function. This state of continuous stress only intensifies the already existing anxiety experienced by the state of mental dysfunctioning. For those who are confused, the present provides little opportunity to avoid the intense anxiety. However, in one's past, a person can illicit any feeling by simply finding the right event. Let me explain further.

We remember things and events from our past because they have attached to them a significant emotional response. This can be demonstrated by the following:

> I want you to relax. After you have read the
> following lines, remove your eyes from the page
> for a moment to concentrate.

Go into your past/
Remember the most positive experience you can/
Relive the event/
Recalling as much about it as you are able/
Experiencing the things that pleased you/

Remove your eyes from the page for a moment to concentrate on
this experience/

What did you encounter? You were probably able to re-experience the original feelings associated with that past event. Whether positive or negative the effect is the same. How many times for no apparent reason have you caught yourself re-calling a bad event or a "hurt" from your past?

If I am void of much emotion save anxiety, then my past becomes my main source for all emotions. Reliving the appropriate event will summon up excitement or elation, happiness or sadness, . . . Again, this need not be a conscious process. The body deals with situations and stress commonly at an unconscious level. The brain is stimulated frequently by the needs of the environment around. For the mentally impaired, past orientation associated with both memory loss and the related depression serves a purpose of touching a range of emotions that may be absent under the present circumstances.

114

3. Occupying Time

The third factor contributing to past orientation is related to sheer boredom.

What happens when you are required to sit for a number of hours at an event that you find boring?

If you can sleep with your eyes open, that is a great talent – don't lose it. Most of us daydream – if we cannot escape physically we will escape mentally.

One of the first courses I taught was pharmacology to a group of 50 first year nursing students. That is a difficult course to get excited about. As a result, I was always on the look-out for that tell tale sign that a student was no longer with me. You know the cues – blank stare, eyes glued to the ceiling, totally unaware of the surroundings. As soon as I spotted that person I would immediately ask "Mary, what do you think about that?" The response was usually one of pure shock and a stammering of "What . . . what?"

What do the mentally impaired do most of the day?

Usually sit. Unless we have something for them to do and are with them encouraging them to do it, they are on their own. With nothing to do comes boredom. The mind wanders. It is better to go into one's past and relive an event than stare at a blank wall for an hour. It simply becomes a way to occupy time. Given that the past is so prevalent to the mentally impaired, going into past events is simple and spontaneous.

4. Providing Familiarity

The forth attribute involves the simple fact that in the present the mentally impaired resident is in a world he does not understand. In the past he can easily re-create one that he does understand. In one's head it is simple to return home, remember family, people you know and things that are familiar. The world in the past is comforting, having associated with it a strong feeling of security. For a while at least, the anxiety and confusion is gone.

This past orientation is accentuated with the mentally impaired by the disease itself. The symptoms of poor recent memory makes the past readily available and alive as if it were now. As a result it is easily accessible, where it can be unconsciously called upon when the emotions of the present become too great and the need to escape or withdraw is the only means to cope.

It can be expected that a good portion of those at the level two in functioning have the potential of being depressed. The mentally impaired may not know what they have lost specifically, but there is a constant feeling that something is missing. This is demonstrated well by the associated feelings of anxiety and the constant "looking for something familiar" in order to control their environment.

Depression and its symptoms will only complicate the ability of the mentally impaired to function. When we discussed secondary factors in chapter two, depression was recognized as having the ability to decrease mental functioning. In this instance when depression is suspected, it is worth treating with an anti-depressive agent. If over a period of six to eight weeks there is an apparent mood elevation, then stay with the drug. If there is no change, then discontinue it.

THE PROCESS OF CONDITIONING

Past orientation can easily "snow ball" into an automatic response, where as soon as the resident sits in a chair and is left alone, he returns to his past. The process that makes it nearly reflex in nature is called "conditioning" – establishing a specific response to a particular stimulus through repeated exposure. Crudely stated, conditioning is the main way to train animals (it requires little cognitive ability) and may be a significant factor in determining some of the behaviours of the mentally impaired.

Past orientation and conditioning can be likened to a child who is a chronic daydreamer. It is not the intention of comparing older adults with children, but it is the process causing chronic daydreaming that demonstrates what may be happening to the mentally impaired.

If you have had contact with a child who is a daydreamer you know the problem well. Such a child will tell you he "can't help it", whenever he sits in a chair "it just happens". The process may be very similar to the following:

> The child is sitting in the classroom
> Whatever the teacher is doing is boring or makes little
>   sense/
> So the child tilts his head up
> Looks to the ceiling
> His mind takes him to another place just for a moment/
>
> When he returns his attention to the present
> His being distracted makes what the teacher is now saying
>   more boring or making less sense/
> So his mind wanders for a longer period/
> When he returns his attention to the present
> His being distracted makes what the teacher is now saying
> More boring or making less sense . . ./

The scenario repeats itself over and over again until the child finds that he only has to sit at a desk and zap . . . he is gone. The desk becomes an anchor, unconsciously associating feelings of boredom each time he sits at it, automatically initiating a daydreaming response. He will soon find as he sits at a desk "it just happens".

We can condition any living thing. Depending on an individual's recall ability, conditioning may be easily applied to the mentally impaired. The more the person is left alone the easier it is to go into the past. After a period all he may have to do is sit and as soon as he is alone he draws into the past.

Combine this concept with the scenario described in chapter two.

> I was in your room doing care from 0730 to 0800 hours.
> I left and returned at 0845 to take you to the bathroom/
> In that period of 45 minutes alone
> It became easy for you to draw into your past/
>
> When I entered at 0845 hours
> I stood over you and asked "Do you have to go to the
>   bathroom?"/
> Did you hear me?

There is no difference between your experience at this time and that of the student in the classroom. You are probably not even aware of my presence let alone what I am saying.

I then take you by the arm and attempt to have you stand/

I am not just taking you from the chair, I am dragging you into my reality. In a matter of seconds, you must move from what you are reliving in your mind to what is happening in the present. In seconds you must determine where you are, who I am and what I am doing. Impossible! Your only logical response to this abrupt change is to become aggressive or resistant as a result of the anxiety created.

We have established that there are two very distinct groups of staff – those who are flexible and very successful with the mentally impaired and those who are task oriented, clinging to a set routine expecting this type of resident to adapt. Staff who are task oriented seem to have the most difficulty. They establish a routine and follow it expecting the resident to maintain the same degree of familiarity and recall. If they have taken a resident to the washroom at 0845 every morning and it is 0845, then that is what will be done. The expectation that the resident knows what is happening results in there being little warning, just action. This lack of sensitivity to the resident's inability to remember who that person is or what she wants can have devastating effects.

Those staff who work "magic", who are most successful in performing their care with the mentally impaired, do so often without being conscious of what makes the difference. The difference is usually in approach. Every contact is made at eye level. Most importantly this staff member will touch the resident as she speaks. No matter the degree of impairment, when a resident is touched, he will generally move his eyes towards you. Making physical contact by placing a hand on the resident's shoulder is an intense stimulus that causes the person to look to the source of that touch. At the moment of eye contact the person is in the "here and now". That level of awareness may only last for seconds but contact is made. Lastly, you speak in a soft tone, asking the resident "Do you have to go to the bathroom?" Allowing the person to internalize what is said, repeating again if necessary and then touching his elbow, you gently guide him up. The probability of successfully having this resident go to the washroom without any major outburst is good.

This approach, no matter how basic, has two very distinct effects. First the resident is being given the opportunity to move from past orientation to present, to become aware of where he is and what is happening. Secondly, he is provided a degree of control over what is being asked of him. Such an approach ensures that the cues the resident is responding to alleviates instead of escalates his anxiety level. In both of these instances what is being established is **rapport**. Rapport is one of the major components of effectively working with the mentally impaired. It provides the resident with an opportunity to feel a degree of security with the person doing the care.

It is important to emphasize that probably many low functioning mentally impaired residents may not understand the content of what is said at any given moment. The words and what they mean may not be as significant as what is perceived.

Imagine:

> You do not understand the following phrase at all
> "Do you have to go to the washroom?"/
> What you see is a smiling face at eye level
> You hear a soft and friendly voice/
> You experience a gentle touch on your arm to encourage
> you to stand/

How would you respond?

Being constantly in a world you do not understand, bombarded by stimuli that is difficult to interpret, you may be left to respond to a person or task based only on the degree of security experienced at the time. Unable to understand what is happening or to rationalize the circumstances, you are left to deal with things as you see them at face value. What is being said may not be as important as how it is done.

Often the key to being successful with the mentally impaired is to stick to the basics. Knowing the experience of this type of resident the best approach is a simple, straightforward one. Given the person's circumstances, it is probably the most logical option.

SEXUAL BEHAVIOUR

In the previous chapter we discussed the impact of labeling as it applied to confusion and aggressive behaviour. There is another label that is very restrictive and damaging. It is called "dirty old man".

Imagine that you have a 79 year old male resident who is mentally impaired. He was married for 57 years. In his marriage, this man was unable to initiate a hug or any such physical contact with his wife. His wife on the other hand met that need for him. She was intuitive to his needs. She provided the hug or physical contact within the relationship. Once she initiated a hug, he would respond accordingly. This man never received this contact from anyone else but his wife. His wife died two years ago, he is now mentally impaired (level two) and living in a long term care facility. When was the last time he was held?

Even if he were cognitively well, this man would have a hard time compensating for the loss of his wife and the subsequent loss of physical contact. He is now further limited by his mental dysfunctioning. For the past two years, given his situation and location, he has experienced significant anxiety and as identified, possibly intense depression. We all know that being under such intense emotional stress, we require physical contact by those around us to provide the security and support needed to survive.

This man is no different. After two years with minimal physical contact, the need for "touch" becomes great. What he unconsciously does to compensate is to touch those in close contact. As we have emphasized again and again – "if you leave the mentally impaired to solve their own problems, the solution will always be inappropriate".

When he touches staff, he can easily be labeled "a dirty old man". When labeled such, how much staff contact does he receive? Probably less. A number of staff may be uncomfortable with his behaviour and avoid him as much as possible. When he is avoided, what does that do to this man's need to be touched? It only intensifies. Therefore, his touching others is increased in order to satisfy that need. That only intensifies the label, which increases the avoidance behaviour, and further increases the need and so on.

Behaviour of the mentally impaired communicates to us their need. In this situation staff have a number of responsibilities.

First, it is obvious that this person has a significant need for physical contact. The responsibility of staff is to be the "aggressor". Not aggressive, but aggressor. That implies that staff must take control of the situation. When in contact with this resident, staff need to initiate touch. Consciously slipping their arm over his shoulder when walking along side him or place a hand over his while standing next to him. In each instance staff must be conscious of providing the needed physical contact. How that person is approached and the manner in which the contact is controlled is important and will be discussed in chapter ten.

The mentally impaired cannot control their behaviour. The responsibility lies with staff. When certain staff are uncomfortable with the touching behaviour presented by specific residents, it is a clue that these staff need direction and support in dealing with this aspect of care. Educational sessions on sexuality and approaching individuals with such overt behaviour whether physical or verbal are mandatory to allow staff to overcome their personal uncomfortableness and develop the necessary professional skills.

Let us examine some sexually explicit situations. By the way, if you are uncomfortable with what is about to be discussed, then you have identified for yourself a need to learn the skills to deal with this behaviour. If you are uncomfortable reading it here, you can only be uncomfortable if you encounter it in your care.

a) Sexual Intercourse

Level two mentally impaired residents are unable to complete sexual intercourse or masturbation. A common comment expressed by a spouse of an Alzheimer's victim is that "My husband will talk about sex, initiate it through petting and fondling, but will never complete it." With such an activity it is not the lack of physical ability that restricts performance, but mental dysfunctioning. Sexual intercourse requires considerable concentration and memory retention. Level two mentally impaired are incapable of maintaining that level of cognitive functioning. When the act is initiated, it is soon forgotten.

The expression of physical sexuality is a natural act. What the mentally impaired lack is the inability to understand when their behaviour is inappropriate and the loss of recent memory to retain any instructions to change it. As the need arises, they respond.

In fact sexual needs are no different than any other needs. We have demonstrated that if the person experiences significant anxiety, he will probably become aggressive or withdraw. If there is a need to urinate, it will be done in what seems to be the right spot for him. Likewise if sexual needs arise, they will be dealt with and then soon forgotten, only to be repeated again as though they never happened. Staff cannot place on the mentally impaired an expectation that they are incapable of comprehending their actions and behaviour when it comes to all tasks of daily living except sexual behaviour. The person is either mentally impaired or cognitively well, he cannot be both.

b) Masturbation

Like intercourse, the dynamics are true with masturbation. The resident may be able to have an erection, fondle himself, but rarely complete to ejaculation. He cannot maintain the concentration and memory retention to complete the act.

Initiating masturbation should not be the issue that concerns staff. Instead it is the location where the behaviour is elicited. The mentally impaired become oblivious to those around them. They are incapable of judging when their behaviour is right or wrong. As a result, you will find certain male or female residents exposing themselves and commence masturbating in some very public places. Staff can attempt as much as they want to stop that behaviour, but they will be unsuccessful. As soon as the behaviour is stopped, it will begin again. The resident forgets what he was just told. The responsibility of the care team is to identify behavioural cues that forewarn that the person is about to begin masturbation (pulling on his zipper, raising her skirt, fondling oneself, etc.). Once those cues are seen it is the responsibility of the staff member who has recognized them (whether nursing, housekeeping, recreation or anyone on that unit) to take the person to his room. Our responsibility is not to stop the behaviour, but to maintain the resident's dignity should the behaviour commence.

c) Relationships: Mentally Impaired Male Resident
with a Mentally Impaired Female Resident

At times you will discover that a specific mentally impaired male resident will always make a bee line to a specific mentally impaired female resident or visa versa. Once sitting together, they will hold hands or begin fondling each other. When a mentally impaired resident always seeks out the same male or female resident there is probably a legitimate reason. Something about that resident either reminds him of his spouse or something about that resident hooks an old memory from the past (a past girl friend). There is no way to keep the two apart unless they are heavily medicated or physically restrained. Neither of these interventions are desirable.

Staff's responsibility is not to intervene in that relationship unless one of the resident's is distressed by the contact or the behaviour becomes inappropriate for the location (exposing each other in the lounge).

A problem can arise when the spouse of one of the resident's is still alive. In this case the spouse must be helped to understand the behaviour – that he/she is not aware of being married and the relationship stems from an association with someone in his past life. This will not always be acceptable to the spouse. She may still find that seeing her husband sit with another woman and holding hands too disturbing. In the case where the wife cannot handle what is happening, then she must take the initiative to decrease the stress created by the situation. She must be encouraged to call the unit a half hour before each visit and instruct other family members to do the same. In that way staff can then separate the two residents before the visit, having one occupied with an activity while the wife is visiting.

This is the same intervention that family would be encouraged to take if a resident had a history of aggressive behaviour. Family would be asked to call before each visit to ensure that it is a "good time". There is no difference in this case. The behaviour is beyond the control of the resident and therefore must be controlled by the care team.

d) Relationships: A Cognitively Well Male Resident
with a Mentally Impaired Female Resident
The circumstances of this situation will dictate the response. If a cognitively well male resident is known to be a very caring and trustworthy gentleman, who initially began a supporting friendship with a level two mentally impaired female resident that turned into an intimate relationship, would you intervene? If the mentally impaired resident responds in a positive manner, I hope you would not intervene. There are no bounds to loving someone. If there were, then a number of existing relationships between well and frail individuals would be in

jeopardy. The key here is that the relationship grew to intimacy and the mentally impaired resident was responding to that person's affection in a positive manner.

In the same vain, we need to discuss another delicate issue. Sometimes a cognitively well male resident targets mentally impaired female residents, and is found fondling, exposing or petting them. In this situation, the attending physician must be asked if he would classify that male resident as mentally incompetent. If the answer is no, then the response is obvious. This behaviour would not be accepted anywhere else. If in the community a person took advantage of someone who was mentally incompetent, he would be charged with sexual assault. A long term care facility has no freedom to have any different expectations, if this situation should arise, then the cognitively well resident must be warned that his behaviour has serious legal ramifications. He must be counseled to assist in stopping his behaviour. If it continues, he must be charged. Some may believe that such an intervention is harsh and unrealistic because the resident is "old". On the contrary, to treat the situation any differently is in contrast to our philosophy of care. First, we are responsible for the physical well being and safety of those under our care. Secondly, we would not allow the mentally impaired to be sexually taken advantage of by a volunteer who was over 65 years just because he is "old". We cannot allow a cognitively well resident leniency because he is a resident. To protect a cognitively well resident from what is normal behaviour just because he is "old" is a stereotypic expectation that the courts would not accept and we cannot tolerate (see ageism in the text Working with the Frail Elderly).

MANIPULATIVE BEHAVIOUR

Can the mentally impaired manipulate?

NO! It is cognitively impossible for a mentally impaired resident to manipulate. In order to manipulate, one requires two pieces of information – you need to know both your options and "cause and effect". This can be demonstrated in the following manner.

If you have children, you have potential manipulators. Again it is not to imply that older adults are like children, but the behaviour demonstrated by children clearly demonstrates the skills needed in order to manipulate.

Imagine:

> You are my mother/
> I am 4 years old/
> I approach you in the kitchen
> "Mom I want to play with you"/
> You respond "Len I am busy right now,
> Why don't you go to your room for a bit and play
> I will be up later to spend some time with you."/

Isn't it remarkable that when you say something like this to your child, if there is anything to break in the house it will probably get broken at that exact moment?

This child knows his options, as well as "cause and effect". One of his options is to return to his room and wait. The other is to return to mom and say "Mom I don't care if you're busy or not, I want to play with you NOW." That would have a specific response. The third option is to get mother's attention by doing something that will require her to "come running". This is better termed "pushing mom's buttons". The decision he makes is at a conscious and well thought–out level.

This child also knows "cause and effect". He is aware there are things he can do that will make mother run to him when he wants her – knock a vase off the table. You can see his mind working even before he knocks over the vase. He looks from one side to the other to see if mother will be in "ear shot" of the noise created when it hits the floor. If mother is not around, the vase may very well stay on the table – why waste energy for little gain – if mother can't hear it hit the floor, he won't get the response he wants.

If you are married follow through with this scenario. If you are not, imagine what the responses may be:

Does your spouse know you?

I don't mean that he knows you the way you may want him to, but does he know when you are hurting emotionally and when to come close? Again it may not be the degree or type of support that you want, but does he respond? Does he know when you are angry and to stay away? Again his response to your anger may not be exactly when and how you want it.

If your answer is no, then you have not looked closely enough at your relationship. When a spouse states "we have nothing in our marriage", it usually means that she does not have the things in her marriage that she wants. You cannot live intimately with someone without gaining a "hand/glove" relationship. Intimate contact every day, each year creates a reflex response neither spouse may be fully aware of. In the years that you are married, subtle cues from one partner to the other are identified and responded to, often at an unconscious level. The manner and degree of response may not be what the other partner expects or wants but there is usually a response. To understand the subtleness of such a long term relationship, just ask a widow what she lost when she lost her husband. She will usually respond that there are things missing now that she was not even conscious of while he was alive.

You are now 78 years old
Mentally impaired
Living on a long term care unit/
Would the staff know you as intimately?

How will they know when you are hurting emotionally?

Only when you cry. You never had to cry for your husband to know that you were hurting. Your husband only had to see the look in your eyes, your expression, or hear a specific tone in your voice to know that there was a problem that required his support.

How will staff know when you are angry?

Only when you become aggressive. Again you rarely had to show your husband such an intense response. He only had to see the subtle cues – the look in your eye, what you did . . ., to know that you were upset.

Am I going to teach you now at 78 years old, mentally impaired, living in a long term care facility how to deal with your emotional needs differently? Impossible! You are left only to respond to your needs at a "gut level". When you are afraid, you call "Mother, mother, mother, . . ." or "Ow, Ow, Ow, . . ." until someone comes to you, talks with you, touches you. Or when you are angry, you bite, spit, kick, until they leave you alone.

The mentally impaired do not manipulate. They do not have the cognitive ability to problem solve in order to decide what options are available to resolve what they are experiencing and have their needs met. Even if told the acceptable options to get the staff's attention or to be left alone, a few moments later they will forget those instructions and resume their previous behaviour. Likewise they do not have the insight to determine cause and effect. Such an analytical process is beyond their ability.

This implies a significant aspect of understanding limitations in care. First a program called behaviour modification is probably one of the cruelest things that could be done to a level two mentally impaired resident. Behaviour modification identifies the behaviour that is unacceptable and ignores it, but rewards the behaviour that is acceptable. You can tell a mentally impaired resident that instead of calling out you want her to do something else. She will respond "Okay". Just as soon as you walk out the door, she will call out again. Remember you cannot teach anything new to a person with poor recent memory retention. She may not understand the instructions given to her on the alternate behaviour; remember what was said; or even be aware that she is repeating herself. You cannot stop the behaviour by simply giving alternate instructions.

Likewise, this reputes those staff who believe she can stop calling out if she wants. This lady knows nothing of cause and effect. She has a need and responds accordingly. She does not even know if calling repeatedly will have any results. She just calls until there is a response. Besides, if she does stop calling, how does she get you?

What the mentally impaired must do is respond to their needs – doing what is necessary given the circumstances experienced at that specific time. A very basic human response.

THE PREMISE FOR CARE

A number of years ago, when I was newly married and first a nurse, my wife and I accompanied 35 mentally handicapped children to Florida for a two week vacation several years in a row. We were the nursing team along with 15 MR Counselors who organized and supervised the function.

Before our first venture, I had little contact with the mentally handicapped. My first two days were the most difficult. Being a newly graduated nurse, I believed I could change the world. In front of me now were a number of severely "retarded" individuals whose behaviours were not unlike what we encounter with the mentally impaired elderly – spastic movements, repetitive speech, and so on.

On the second day, I finally dragged aside an MR Counselor who had considerable experience with this clientele. I said to her "Can't you see these children are having problems – considerable difficulty in their movements and speech? Why don't you do something to help them correct that?" I learned more on how to deal with our clientele from that person than from anyone else since.

She responded, "These children are mentally handicapped due to brain damage. There is nothing I can do to reverse the brain damage, therefore there is nothing I can do to stop the symptoms. My job is to look beyond the symptoms to see what is left of the person and then provide to the part that remains the greatest quality of life I can."

In caring for the mentally impaired elderly we unfortunately seem to place our emphasis more on the symptoms, than the person. The brain damage experienced by the mentally impaired cannot be reversed, nor can it be stalled. We have been charged with the responsibility of providing to this person the highest level of quality of life possible. Hence the premise for Supportive Therapy – identifying his strengths and maintaining them, his limitations and compensating for them.

This means taking risks at times. No approach, environment or intervention works the same way all of the time for all of those who are mentally impaired. Our challenge is to determine which is the effective intervention during each moment of contact.

No matter what our approach with the mentally impaired, there can be positive and negative consequences experienced. But not to take a risk, not to search for what is the most appropriate for this individual is to shelter that person in a cocoon, a process that will return us to custodial care and remove from him any quality of life.

I was asked to assess a unit housing a number of mentally impaired residents that demonstrated a great deal of disruptive wandering behaviour. Based on my initial assessment of the unit, the lounge seemed to be the source of most of the problems. I established my plan of action – I would sit in the resident's lounge to see how long I could last before I wanted to wander. The best vantage point was a two seated couch against one wall. One of the residents, a mentally impaired gentleman occupied one side of the couch. He was slumped over, staring at the floor. (Staff later shared with me that this was his normal posture and he was usually expressionless and rarely communicated). I had no intention of maintaining a conversation with this man, only to assess the lounge. When I sat I said "hello" and then proceeded to watch the lounge.

After 15 minutes of my sitting next to him, the man turned and stared at me. He stared for a good 5 minutes until he said "potatoes". I repeated to him "potatoes". For the next 15 minutes this man talked to me about his potato farm of 40 years ago – who worked on it, the problems he had, the money he made or lost, etc. During our conversation there was a dramatic shift in this man's posture and expression. He now sat erect, his face beamed and he grinned from ear-to-ear during the entire time we discussed his farm.

That was the end of my day, so I said good-bye to my new acquaintance and left the unit. I returned the next morning. When I walked past the nurse's station, I was accosted by the head nurse.

She said to me "What did you do to that man last night?"

I said "I don't know, what did I do?"
"I don't know what you did either, but when you left last night, that resident got up, got a hold of a waste paper basket and spent 4 hours wandering the unit looking for his potatoes. Don't do it again!"

I said "Just a minute, was he a behavioural problem during that time? Was he disruptive, disturbing others?"
She responded "No, he wasn't disturbing anyone. The problem was he wouldn't eat when he was supposed to eat, he wouldn't wash when he was supposed to wash and he wouldn't go to sleep when he normally does."

I asked, "After the four hours, did he eat, did he wash and did he go to bed?"

She answered "Yes, he did."

And I returned, "What was the problem?"

If this nurse meant that I was not to allow this gentleman to experience anything positive because he disrupted her routine, then dig a hole and put him in it. Quality of life is more than physical care. No matter what you do with the mentally impaired, whether positive or negative, it will have consequences. If you elicit from a mentally impaired individual something positive, then it may bring back memories and that will elicit a change in behaviour. Likewise, if you intensify the resident's anxiety level, you will elicit agitation or wandering.

The goal of care is more complex than any medical model that deals with the symptoms of the disease. We have been charged with making the remainder of this person's life the most positive possible, given the limitations experienced. That may require our taking the person's symptoms and doing little more than making them tolerable to ourselves who do the care and the other residents who must live with him. To emphasize only the physical aspects of this person's life brings us back to the days of custodial care, which is a frustrating environment for both the staff and the resident.

Our approach to care is one of risk taking – attempting something, if it works, stay with it. If it doesn't, set it aside and move on to something else. Like life, there is nothing more insignificant than emphasizing only one need, only one part of what gives life meaning. We deal with every part of this person for the rest of his life, for one goal only – quality of life.

SUMMARY

If I were dying from terminal cancer and experiencing excruciating pain, your telling me that I have no pain, does not make it go away. Likewise, if I am mentally impaired, your believing that I should understand or be able to act "normal", does not mean that my impairment goes away.

One very important question that must be asked when discussing resident behaviour is:

Is that person cognitively well or mentally impaired?

You cannot be both. If mentally impaired, then do not imply ability and understanding that the person cannot possess.

Caring for the mentally impaired is not an easy job. Nor is it a simple process to always be objective, constantly placing oneself behind the eyes of this resident. There are times when those skills of being objective and empathetic are strained to their limit. It takes a "special" staff to work with such a client experiencing "special" needs.

To be effective in providing care we must have clearly defined and enforced programs specifically geared to this individual and his limitations. Developing and implementing the most appropriate programming for the specific needs of this individual. If the challenge is met, we will ensure for this resident that he will achieve the highest level of quality of life, living in an environment that is supportive – compensating for his limitations and enhancing his strengths.

Chapter Seven

The Care Process

Once one understands the progressive and deteriorative nature of Alzheimer's or Multiple Infarct diseases, it is easy to understand the misconception that little can be done with this clientele. It is true nothing can be done to arrest or cure the mental impairment, but a great deal can be done to provide the remainder of this person's life with the greatest degree of quality possible.

The basis of the Supportive Therapy approach is – identifying for that person his strengths and maintaining them; identifying his limitations and compensating for them. Such an approach requires an array of programming options, given the individuality of symptoms and limitations experienced by the client.

The following is an overview of those options. If you work in a long term care setting, complete this questionnaire as an evaluation mechanism to determine the strengths and weakness within your own unit. If you do not work in such an area, read it through and think of it as an overview of the interventions to be discussed in the following chapters.

EVALUATING THE CARE PROCESS AVAILABLE FOR THE MENTALLY IMPAIRED RESIDENT

The following is an overview of many of the components required to successfully provide care to the mentally impaired elderly in long term care facilities. To determine the strengths and weaknesses of your facility in this area, check the appropriate number next to each statement:

    1. In place and working
    2. In place but needs further development or is not
          consistent
    3. Non−existent

PHILOSOPHY

_ _ _ 1. The philosophy in caring for the mentally impaired establishes that these residents are to be treated as "normal" functioning adults without expectations of "normal" behaviour.

_ _ _ 2. Periodic aggressive or resistive outbursts are acceptable behaviour, understanding that for some mentally impaired this is the only means to communicate one's frustration with the circumstances encountered.

_ _ _ 3. Physical contact (touching, holding, hugging, etc.) is stressed – staff are encouraged to maintain touch as a form of communicating to residents beyond times of performing basic care tasks.

_ _ _ 4. Staff have accepted that certain behaviours (i.e. wandering, repetitive behaviours, etc.) do not require intervention unless they create negative consequences.

_ _ _ 5. The cognitively well residents in contact with the mentally impaired are given directions on what to expect when encountering such a resident and how to deal with common problems.

1 2 3

ADMISSION

_ _ _ 1. A pre–admission meeting is held, allowing a representative of those staff who will be performing the care to meet and assess the potential resident. If an admission candidate is in hospital, a staff member from the admitting unit is required to visit the hospital to gain as much information as possible regarding the care process and routines already established.

_ _ _ 2. Where possible, the new resident and his or her family are gradually introduced to the unit prior to admission by establishing daily visits where meals and programs can be observed or participated in.

_ _ _ 3. Families are given an admission package outlining their role, philosophy of care for the mentally impaired resident, programs involved, etc.

_ _ _ 4. Families are given a questionnaire on admission for them to outline specific care issues already encountered – likes, dislikes, routines, abilities, how behavioural problems have been dealt with to this point, etc.

_ _ _ 5. During the first three days of admission, the new resident is assigned to the same staff member on each shift to decrease the amount of change encountered and provide consistency in approach and care.

_ _ _ 6. Basic care is only performed during the first few days of admission – bath, detailed assessment, activity involvement, etc. are withheld until a degree of familiarity is gained by the resident to the unit and staff.

_ _ _ 7. During the first few days of admission, the new resident is allowed time away from other residents and the routine of the unit.

_ _ _ 8. A meeting is held with family and staff who have cared for the new resident shortly after admission to determine any noted changes and provide adjustment and direction to the care process.

_ _ _ 9. The admission criteria accepts the limits of both our environment and our staff by barring the general admission of expsychiatric patients unless a trial period can be negotiated with the referring agency, guaranteeing the individual will be returned if he/she cannot be cared for safely in our environment.

1 2 3   **ENVIRONMENT**

__ __ __   1. Environmental cuing (colour coding and locator signs) is used to assist the resident to find specific areas on the unit.

__ __ __   2. Anchoring is employed to assist the resident to identify specific areas on the unit (i.e personal bedspread on their bed, specific decor on their door, etc.).

__ __ __   3. The environment looks "normal", assisting the resident to function by hooking "old memory" – dining room looks like a dining room, lounge like a living room, etc.

__ __ __   4. There are areas available that allow the mentally impaired and cognitively well residents to be separate.

__ __ __   5. There is a specific and clearly defined wandering path available to the mentally impaired residents.

__ __ __   6. Exit doors accessible to the wanderer are secured (magnetic or combination locking system) to allow the wanderer free and safe wandering.

__ __ __   7. There is a secured courtyard that allows free access to the outside by all residents.

__ __ __   8. Things familiar to the resident's past are accessible in his/her room.

__ __ __   9. All resident bedrooms housing the mentally impaired are private occupancy only.

__ __ __   10. Multiple small sitting areas are available for those residents who cannot handle stress or distractions.

__ __ __   11. Reality reinforcement is employed – i.e. cuing in the environment identifies to the resident needed

135

information – staff name tags, clocks, calendars, etc.

1 2 3

PROGRAMS

1. Activity programs available to the mentally impaired are very distinct from programs available to other residents.

2. The activity department is required to maintain a list of mentally impaired residents and the programs each is involved in.

3. Sensory stimulation is employed by nursing, recreation and dietary department as an ongoing program.

4. There are adequately supervised large group activities for all mentally impaired residents.

5. There are a variety of small group activities geared to all levels of resident functioning.

6. There are regular outings for all mentally impaired residents.

7. Things of normal life are available – pets, plants, children, magazines, newspapers, radio, TV., etc.

8. Chores are available to all residents, geared to the individual's functioning level – i.e. cleaning glasses, setting tables, folding linen, etc.

9. Activity equipment is available on the unit for any staff, volunteer or family to use at any time.

1 2 3

CARE

1. Care is flexible, staff adjust their care in consideration of the circumstances and behaviour encountered with a resident at any one time –

bathing, meals, etc. – no routine other than the routine of the specific resident is crucial.

2. A form of primary care exists where specific staff are responsible for a specific number of residents over a period of time even though physical care on the unit is completed as a team function.

3. The care team involves various departments – nursing, housekeeping, dietary and supportive staff, with opportunities for input from all other departments and family as well.

4. Staff are involved in a process of care analysis where all staff on the unit discuss the needs of each resident and the best direction for care.

5. The assignment of staff ensures that for every full time staff working in an area, there is the same part time staff replacing him/her each week.

6. There is an effective care plan in place providing staff with the specifics of a resident's routine, guidelines on what is commonly done by the full time staff working with that individual, etc.

7. A detailed outline of the care plan accompanies any mentally impaired resident transferred to hospital, along with the name of a facility contact person that hospital staff can call should problems in care occur.

8. Family are considered an integral part of the care process, being informed of any changes in condition or care, and utilized to augment the care provided.

9. The care plan for the mentally impaired resident is distinct from those involving the cognitively well resident, emphasizing the psychological and behavioural issues rather than the physical.

1 2 3   **ASSESSMENT**
— — —   1. Any noted change in a resident's behaviour or
               functioning initiates assessment.

— — —   2. Functional assessments are completed on all
               residents at regular intervals.

— — —   3. All staff (R.N., R.N.A., aides, recreation staff,
               etc.) are involved in the assessment process.

— — —   4. The assessment process includes: a functional
               assessment (i.e 24 hour profile), mental status (i.e
               Kingston Dementia Scale), medical, medication
               review, detailed history, environmental assessment
               and psychological profile.

— — —   5. Staff are involved in continually outlining the
               history of this resident as pieces of information are
               obtained. A form, at the front of the chart allows
               staff from all departments to add new information.

— — —   6. Each resident is assessed to determine the
               appropriateness of any environmental cues used in
               the facility – name bar, colour coding, picture, etc.

— — —   7. A process of ongoing assessment, observing
               subtle cues from a specific resident in order to
               adjust care, is taught to all staff.

1 2 3   **DRUGS & RESTRAINTS**
— — —   1. Drugs are administered for resident behavioural
               problems only when required, after other means are
               attempted to deal with the issue, and as a stop gap
               if possible until circumstances change.

— — —   2. A Three Month Drug Review requires an
               automatic stop order on all drugs every three
               months, where each drug recorded is treated as a
               new order and the rationale for that drug written on
               the Doctor's Progress Notes.

_____ 3. Non−life maintenance drugs (sedations, sleeping pills, etc.) are subject to a trial period of non−use when the initiating behaviour or circumstance is no longer obvious, the dosage is decreased or the drug completely stopped for three weeks with a backup sedation available should problems occur.

_____ 4. All devices restricting the mobility of a resident are considered restraints. A restraint policy exists requiring the team (including the physician) to decide whether any restraint is to be used on a specific resident, and outlines precautions to be taken during the time the restraint is applied to the resident.

_____ 5. Residents who are chronically physically violent – a threat to the safety of other residents and staff, regardless of the interventions attempted by staff – are transferred to the local hospital for proper placement.

_____ 6. A policy exists that outlines to all staff the steps that must be taken to conduct a search when a resident wanders from the building.

1 2 3   **STAFF**
_____ 1. All staff have been polled to identify those who do not wish to work with mentally impaired residents. Those staff are not assigned to that level of care if at all possible.

_____ 2. Full and part time staff working with the mentally impaired are consistent, keeping to a minimum the number of staff in contact with an individual resident in a 7 day period.

_____ 3. Each department is responsible to monitor and develop programming for the mentally impaired residents in the building – recreation, adjuvant, social services (where applicable), etc.

___ ___ 4. Staff in contact with the mentally impaired have been trained to understand the process of the disease affecting this resident, possible behaviours that may be encountered and the appropriate interventions to be undertaken.

___ ___ 5. Staff responsible for the care of the mentally impaired residents in the building have direct input into decisions regarding that care, the environment in which these residents live and the programs affecting care.

___ ___ 6. There is a designated "Special Care Coordinator" who has the responsibility to ensure that the mentally impaired residents in the building receive the same quality of life and advantages as other residents in the building.

___ ___ 7. A staff member who has difficulty performing care with a specific resident is not assigned that resident (instances where the resident is a problem to a number of staff or one staff member has problems with a number of residents are dealt with individually).

___ ___ 8. A distinct support system exists for those staff working with the mentally impaired where time, break periods and routines can be adjusted given the circumstances experienced on a specific day.

1 2 3

FAMILY

___ ___ 1. Family and significant others are considered part of the care process and are given the needed direction on their involvement in the care and activities of the resident.

___ ___ 2. Family nights are arranged regularly through the year to allow families the opportunity to meet with other families of mentally impaired residents, to learn about the disease process, programming options, the family's role and also provide families

140

the chance to share with each other their feelings and experiences.

___ ___ 3. All family members of Alzheimer's victims (whether they are regular visitors or not) are referred to the local Alzheimer's Society for assistance and provided a list of available resource texts.

___ ___ 4. Families are notified in advance (through direct phone call, letter or a family bulletin board located in the facility) of any activities or outings scheduled for the mentally impaired residents in which family can participate.

___ ___ 5. Families are provided the name of a contact person at the local Family and Children Counselling Agency to assist in dealing with the emotional issues that have risen through the course of the disease of their loved one.

___ ___ 6. The expertise of those families who have cared for a mentally impaired family member is recognized and these families are encouraged to volunteer their services to assist in programs available in the building.

1 2 3

VOLUNTEERS

___ ___ 1. All volunteers are prepared for the possible behaviours they may encounter from the mentally impaired and the best approaches to be taken.

___ ___ 2. All volunteers available to the home are polled to identify those who would like to work with the mentally impaired directly and in what capacity.

___ ___ 3. Volunteers who are asked to work with the mentally impaired directly have been trained to understand the resident's behaviour and the most appropriate interventions and approaches to be taken.

_____ 4. All volunteers dealing with the mentally impaired are buddied with the staff member who best knows the resident in order to assist in any problems that may be encountered.

1 2 3
_____
RESOURCES
1. The care team has contacts with outside agencies and professionals for consultation when dealing with psychiatric problems.

_____ 2. All staff are encouraged to maintain their expertise by participating in training opportunities outside of the facility.

_____ 3. Staff visit other facilities involved in caring for the mentally impaired to share and learn further skills.

_____ 4. The facility has a mandate to share its developments and accomplishments by submitting material to association publications or appropriate journals.

1 2 3
_____
AUXILIARY PROGRAMS
1. A Day Program is available within the facility for the mentally impaired living in the community.

_____ 2. A Respite or Vacation Care program for the mentally impaired living with family in the community is in place and well advertised.

_____ 3. The facility is utilized as a resource centre for family caring for mentally impaired individuals living in the community, encouraging them to call to gain information and assistance.

_____ 4. The facility has offered itself as a base for the local Alzheimer's Society or as a location to hold periodic meetings.

SUMMARY

We are defining a specialty that is as challenging as any in the health care field. All of the interventions and concepts presented are worthwhile and practical mechanisms for effectively caring for the mentally impaired. The immediate response to this overview is that we do not have the resources, time or expertise to implement what is suggested.

This is a developing industry and one that continues to evolve. Your task is to decide which of these exists and is working well in your facility and which is the priority for implementation at this time. The "magic" possessed by some individuals or some facilities in their success in caring for the mentally impaired is based totally on the energies they have invested to ensure such interventions are adapted to their environment and their resources.

As we discuss the options in care, your responsibility lies in determining which can best be adopted or implemented in the setting in which you work, in order for your facility and staff to provide the most supportive care for those living within.

Chapter Eight

Programming

We have spent considerable time discussing the concept of Supportive Therapy. What we have identified to this point can now be summarized into very specific objectives concerning the care process and environment. These objectives include:

1. Providing security and safety for the wandering resident.
2. Providing the mentally impaired with consistency in routines and staff.
3. Establishing a philosophy specific to the needs of the mentally impaired.
4. Having a specific care process that involves analysis and assessment of cognitive functioning, with an admission and discharge procedure specific to the unit.
5. Having available specific social and activity programs geared to cognitive functioning level.
6. Having staff skilled in working with the mentally impaired in the area of: approach, communication, assessment and understanding.
7. Having a mechanism to define the individual vulnerability of each resident.
8. Having an environment that is adapted to the needs of the clientele.

These objectives comprise the foundation for programming for the mentally impaired that will be presented in the following chapters. Let us first begin in this chapter by discussing the possible need for a specialized unit, and then admission.

INTEGRATION VERSUS AUTONOMY

There has been considerable controversy whether the mentally impaired resident should be on the same unit as the cognitively well/physically disabled resident or located on a separate unit with like residents. If the question is simply one of segregation, without the provision of appropriate supports, then the answer is a simple one – no! Segregation, for the sake of segregation alone, has significant negative connotations that are well merited.

To segregate is to take from view or remove from sight. If that is the intention of such a unit then it should never be considered. Without a well–structured plan of action and clear–cut guidelines, such a unit can easily become a "dumping ground" – a location where any "difficult" resident is placed to prevent him from disturbing others. Such a setting merely becomes a warehouse. Unfortunately some facilities have such a unit – very little programming, no admission or discharge criteria, untrained staff and so on. These are the ones that give autonomous units for the mentally impaired an undeserved reputation.

Most facilities employ a form of segregation to some degree or another even though they may not have a separate unit for the mentally impaired. It is common to find many residents located on specific units or floors based on need and functioning. Level two mentally impaired residents who have a tendency to wander are often placed on the second floor, to make it more difficult to wander out the front door and leave the building. Units are often divided where bed care residents are located on one floor or unit, ambulatory/well residents on another and so on. By the way, if the facility doesn't take these steps to place the mentally impaired resident in one area or on one unit, then usually the residents who are cognitively well will employ some form of segregation.

If a unit is totally integrated, you will commonly discover many cognitively well residents sitting in the lounge in the front lobby, in an activity room or in their room in order to stay away from "those crazy people" as many of the mentally impaired are called.

A unit for the mentally impaired is selective in who it serves. The level one mentally impaired, the individual who is aware there is a problem and is still able to function with minimal supports, does not require such a specialized setting. Likewise level three of functioning, or those who are severely impaired both mentally and physically, do not require such a unit. A unit for the mentally impaired is specifically intended for the mentally impaired at level two of functioning – those who are physically well, experiencing a considerable degree of impairment and require specific and intense supports.

Those in level two of functioning require a totally autonomous setting – one that places such a resident in a controlled environment suitable to his functioning level. It is a setting that recognizes and supports this resident in the three areas of his greatest vulnerability:

1. The Environment

This is the resident who does not deal well with excessive stimuli, change and noise. If the environment in which he lives lacks controls in these areas, his anxiety level is easily intensified, actively affecting his cognitive functioning, increasing the tendency for an aggressive or resistive response or uncontrolled wandering behaviour.

2. Other Residents

The mentally impaired are very vulnerable when interacting with cognitively well residents.

You are cognitively well, physically disabled/
I am mentally impaired/
It is the 17th time this morning
I have been in your room going through your things/

How will you respond?

Your anger to this frequent intrusion will be vented by raising your voice and shouting. That not only results in an agitated response from myself, but will influence staff's effectiveness in their providing care to me for the rest of the day. As stated earlier, once my anxiety level is elevated, my functioning ability may be effected throughout the next two shifts.

Your anger may even be great enough that you give me a shove as I walk through the door. Now you have a mentally impaired resident with a broken hip.

3. Again Other Residents

Likewise the cognitively well residents are very vulnerable in their interactions with the mentally impaired.

I have entered your room 17 times/
In my mind all of your things are mine/
I do not understand why you are telling me to get away
from my things/

Now you have the potential of a cognitively well resident experiencing a broken hip, as he argues with a mentally impaired resident.

Establishing a specialized unit for the mentally impaired is much more than just "segregating". An autonomous unit for the mentally impaired emphasizes one fundamental concept – this type of resident is no longer "normal" in an environment that is not "normal". This person could not function in his home where he lived for years, nor with his spouse or family who he has known all of his life. Without a specialized unit, how is he able to function in our environment where the stimuli fluctuates and faces change frequently?

Success in caring for the mentally impaired is enhanced when the environment is constant and the stimuli is low. Such an approach cannot be easily achieved unless programming for this type of resident is clearly defined and constantly enforced.

Autonomous units for the mentally impaired are often called Special Care or Protective Units. They have clearly defined objectives that make them supportive to the special needs of the mentally impaired.

The goal of these units is to provide the mentally impaired with a suitable environment with the least amount of stimuli and the greatest degree of consistency. Residents on such a unit are encouraged to be involved in programs with other residents in the rest of the building, but that involvement is well planned with the needed supports in place.

Much of what will be discussed from this point on will involve programming for the mentally impaired regardless of their location. In the text "Guide to Caring For The Mentally Impaired Elderly", Ontario Association of Homes For The Aged, Metheun Publishing, 1985 (previously titled "Does It Really Matter If Its Tuesday?") such a unit and the components necessary to make it successful are discussed. The intention of this book is to examine the care issues involved in dealing with the mentally impaired elderly whether they are living on an autonomous unit or an integrated one.

Before leaving this topic of integration versus autonomy, it is important to establish one other factor that reinforces the need to consider such a unit.

> I would like you to identify a mentally impaired resident
>   under your care/
> One who wanders or is easily agitated/
> Take that person home with you
> Where you are required to live with that individual
> Twenty–four hours per day/
> Seven days a week/
> For a period of three months/
> Without any break/
>
> How would you be at the end of the three month period?

It is one thing to care for such an individual and be able to leave the unit after an eight hour shift. It is another to have to live with a person who is mentally impaired, easily agitated or wanders constantly. Isn't that what we expect of our cognitively well residents on an integrated unit. If the family of a mentally impaired resident couldn't cope with that person's behaviour at home, how can we expect our cognitively well residents to cope in their home?

Our cognitively well/physically disabled residents are struggling themselves to establish a quality of life given their circumstances (refer to "Working With The Frail Elderly: Beyond The Physical Disability"), let alone understand and cope with the behaviours of the wandering mentally impaired. For the sake of both the mentally impaired and the cognitively well residents, an autonomous unit becomes a realistic option.

ADMISSION

As will be discussed, admission to long term care is a complex process that must be well planned. Without doing so, considerable turmoil will be experienced by the newly admitted mentally impaired individual, their family and the staff involved. In long term care, there is little need for the so called "emergency admissions" – a crisis situation that requires the new admission to be admitted now without any of the preliminary work–up and

148

planning. Such crisis intervention is the role of the hospital, not a long term care facility. Our staffing and resources are not adequate to handle such a quick transition and the consequences of such a rescue are usually disastrous for all concerned.

To understand the impact of admission, we need to return to a scenario outlined in chapter one.

> You were blindfolded and had ear plugs placed in your
> ears/
> Transported to a location you did not know
> The blindfold and ear plugs were removed/
> You were left there/
> Not knowing anyone
> Not understanding what was said to you
> Not being able to read and interpret any signs around you/

That scenario closely portrays the experience of a mentally impaired individual being admitted to a long term care facility.

The first week of admission is a crucial period for many new residents who are mentally impaired. That period can be a time where this person establishes either a state of security or one of intense fear. If within the first few days of arriving on the unit, a new admission with limited mental ability is expected to respond appropriately to:

– a bath given by someone who is not familiar in an
  environment that is unknown
– sleep the first few nights in a room that now has one or more
  roommates who are not known and whose behaviour
  may not be understood
– eat in a dining room that has possibly 30 other people eating,
  where noise and movement is constant
– function in a setting that has a maze of rooms
– relate immediately to unfamiliar people performing intimate
  care tasks whose faces change every 8 hours

Indeed, if this is the case, then the expectations are in error.

The mentally impaired are admitted to long term care for one very specific reason. They could no longer cope living in their own home that they have known for years or with a spouse or family around who they have associated with most of their life. How can that same person be expected to successfully function within hours of being admitted to a unit that has 30 or more residents living within it, some of whom themselves are severely impaired physically, mentally or both? Where he is confronted by a large living space, where all rooms look the same, and the lounge and dining room do not resemble home and the noise level and commotion is always high and constant? A unit where the faces of those who do the care change every eight hours, every day of the week? For that new resident, the fear level must be intense.

A person who is cognitively well can be prepared and supported through the entire admission process. Admission is usually discussed with that person well in advance of the application being made. There is an opportunity for the cognitively well to express their concerns and fears, to clarify issues that are not understood, to visit the facility in advance and familiarize himself with the surroundings, to meet some of the staff that may be performing his care. On the day of admission he can be supported by other residents, staff and family; be familiarized with his surroundings again by touring the unit; have written instructions and routines left at his bedside to help him remember what must be done and when; have the opportunity to talk to others as needed about his fears and helped as often as needed with the transition. There are no such luxuries in preparing the mentally impaired individual for admission.

No matter what is said prior to that day, it will be forgotten. No matter what is discussed on the way to the facility, it will be forgotten. No matter what steps are taken to orientate this person to the people and surroundings, they will be forgotten. All that will be experienced is an intense confusion to what is happening, a bombarding of stimuli in a very short period of time. The first few days of admission can only create for the mentally impaired a feeling of being out of control. Their anxiety is increased to a panic level. In that state of emotional saturation, mental functioning is decreased. Simple tasks that were easily done the day before entering the facility will be temporarily lost. The only response can be of wandering or becoming aggressive.

Admission to long term care for the mentally impaired can aptly be called Transition Shock. It is a period of time where the person experiences so much change in such a short period that their abilities decrease and their level of dysfunctioning increases. This is well supported by the frequent comments of family of new admissions. They will often state shortly after admitting their loved one to a long term care facility "I never realized that my mother was so confused." What they are witnessing is mother's response to dramatic change.

The first experiences of a new admission could dictate his response to that unit for an extended period of time. If within the first week there is a constant sense of panic, that emotional distress and fear in some may last for a considerable period of time. It could easily take a month for a newly admitted mentally impaired resident to gain any familiarity to the smallest aspects of the unit, care and the people performing it. In fact the panic level initiated during the first few days of admission could take a year for it to subside and for some it may never be lessened.

This is not to imply that making the admission process more sensitive to the needs of the mentally impaired will eliminate all aggressive and wandering behaviour of new residents. As we have stated there is no one intervention that will stop all of the symptoms of the mentally impaired. A supportive admission process does lessen the dramatic behavioural swings encountered, making admission a more tolerable experience for the resident who must live through it, for the family who must witness it and for the staff who are required to cope with it.

The responsibility of the unit is to make that first week of admission a gradual process of change. The steps taken at that time will decrease the upheaval and problems encountered. To discuss these steps, we need to divide the admission process into three areas:

1. Introductory Period
2. Transition Period
3. Orientation Period

1. Admission –The Introductory Period

The Introductory Period is the time before admission. Knowing this resident cannot be prepared for admission in advance, this period of time allows the care team and family an opportunity to prepare. This is when the new resident and his family are required to make contact in advance with the unit and the staff who will possibly do the care. It also provides members of the care team the opportunity to meet this resident before admission to gain some critical information that cannot be easily obtained by any pre–assessment forms.

a) Pre–admission Meeting

Pre–admission meetings of perspective residents is not new for most facilities. Unfortunately many facilities limit that meeting to only a select few participants from the facility. The pre–admission meeting must not only include the charge nurse of the unit where this new admission will most likely be placed, but also a direct line representative of that care team. The goal of this contact is to establish some direction on what needs to be done or not done during the first few days of admission. It also provides an opportunity for the resident and his family to meet someone who will possibly be providing that care.

If the new resident is in hospital prior to admission and unable to attend the pre–admission meeting, it is important that the charge nurse and/or staff member from the unit have the opportunity to visit the potential resident in that setting. This will allow staff the opportunity to talk personally with hospital personnel who have performed much of this individual's care. This meeting provides the chance to identify what has already been found successful and what should be avoided.

The pre–admission meeting provides staff the opportunity to ask specific questions of issues very relevant to their day–to–day care routines. An assessment form may indicate that this person is incontinent periodically. Direct line staff would be more specific in the information asked of family "How do you know when your mother has to go to the bathroom?" The pre–admission profile sheets may indicate that this new resident resists taking medication. Staff would ask "Which jam does your mother like to eat?", allowing them the opportunity to successfully camouflage the drugs given. The examples of specific data that would be relevant to staff in those first few days are many. If this information is not gained before admission, there is no question that it will be discovered days after admission. Through trial and error staff in that first week will learn what they must do or must not do. Unfortunately, discovering the information after admission is not only a waste of time and energy, but it comes at the expense of the new admission. Without having an opportunity to gain the individualized data prior to admission, staff are unable to respond to this person's needs specifically, resulting in major behavioural swings that are difficult to control.

b) Preparing for the Admission Time

Once staff have the opportunity to make the base line data relevant to their needs on the unit, they can then use the pre-admission meeting to outline to the family further steps in the admission process – admission time, articles available, room arrangement, etc. This is not a haphazard scheduling, nor a standard format. It must be individualized to each admission.

The time of day of any admission must be set by the staff of the unit. Admission should be at a time when the unit is experiencing the least amount of activity. When the unit is at a low activity level it decreases the amount of bombarding of stimuli this new resident is subjected to during the first few hours on the unit. That alone will have a significant calming effect on this person's fear level. You can imagine the results if this new admission is first introduced to the unit at its most chaotic time. There is nothing more frustrating than to see a mentally impaired individual admitted in the morning when staff are engulfed in the routines of the unit and little attention can be given him or his family during those first few trying hours. Admission time must be when staff can realistically focus their attention on this person.

c) Personal Belongings

It is also important at the pre-admission meeting to identify with family the personal articles of the new admission that they intend to bring in and how they should be arranged in that person's room. It is important that these details be discussed in advance of admission and family be instructed that these articles arrive a few hours before admission.

Having the person's articles arrive at the same time as he is admitted is of little value. Usually the articles are whisked away to be labeled and the person does not get them until later that day or even the next day. Familiar articles must be in place before the resident walks onto the unit. In this way, the new resident sees a room that already has a degree of familiarity attached to it, decreasing much of the transition anxiety by eliminating some of the foreign element.

d) Preparing for the Day

The pre–admission meeting also allows staff to establish with family what meal the new resident would best relate to on the first day as well as the appropriate activity (something the new resident is used to doing) the family, new resident and staff can be involved in for the first afternoon. The more information that can be obtained to plan that first day, the more effective staff will be in decreasing the transition shock felt by the resident.

Finally, staff must identify for family the best and worse times for them to leave the unit on that first day of admission as well. New families will not know the busy or slack times during the shift. Sometimes they feel it is best to just drop dad off and leave. On the contrary, it must be stressed with family that their participation in settling their father on that day is crucial to the admission process. Likewise, family must be told the time that they can walk off the unit and leave dad behind. It is important for staff to outline their normal schedule for that shift and the next. Family have the tendency to want to leave when the unit is busy. They often believe that they are "in the way" if they stay. On the contrary, staff must instruct the family that they expect the opposite. Telling family that the staff need them to stay when the unit is the busiest and staff are not able to provide their parent any extra time, and to leave when the unit is the least busy so that staff can have a better opportunity to be free to occupy mother as the family leave.

e) Pre–Visits

Pre–visits can be arranged prior to admission. This can be during the day, evening or on weekends, whichever time is best for family. The pre–visit provides an opportunity to bring the potential resident in a few days prior to admission for a meal or to attend a specific function.

Advance contact with the unit will give staff and family an indication of some of the problems that may be experienced on admission day. Mother's reaction to the environment, the stimuli, other residents, the activities, etc. can be noted and plans made in advance on how to deal with those issues on the upcoming day.

It is important that family be part of this process to decrease their fear about the facility and define their role in this resident's care. The more this can be achieved in advance, the more apt family are to remain an integral part of this resident's life after admission.

2. Admission – The Transition Period

a) Staff Support
The transition period is the first shift when the new resident is admitted. During the first few hours when that new resident is on the unit, it is important that a staff member be relieved from other duties in order that she may be solely assigned to this new individual and his family. That suggestion usually raises eyebrows of managers and staff from some facilities.

To accomplish this, it is not necessary for the facility to call in an extra staff member for an added eight hour shift or to leave the unit short staffed. What is required is adding a four hour casual shift at the time of admission. The role of this casual worker is to relieve a full time staff member from her duties, allowing the permanent staff member time to spend the added time with the new resident.

A common comment made by some staff to such a suggestion is that the budget could not afford the cost of an extra 4 hours. We need to examine this further before this option is negated on the grounds of cost. First, it is important to identify the number of yearly admissions of mentally impaired individuals at level two functioning level.

Admissions to long term care of a level two functioning ability in an average size facility would be no more than two on average each month. Remember that is an average. Some months it may be more and other months less. Also remember that number does not include new admissions representing other levels of functioning and other abilities. The need for added staff is not necessary when admitting individuals at level one and three of mental dysfunctioning and those who are cognitively well/physically disabled.

Two admissions per month of level two translates into 24 half shifts per year or a total of 12 full shifts. If converted to hours paid at a pay rate of $13.00 per hour (personal care worker or nurse's aide) that translates to a yearly cost of $1248.00. That is a minuscule amount of any budget. The benefits of such an investment far out ways the minimal costs. Unfortunately even that amount will be resisted in some facilities who neither understand the need for such support or manage by a "nickel/dime" mentality. They look only to immediate costs rather than the actual investment of worker hours if the support is not provided.

b) Staff Responsibilities

The staff member assigned to this new resident for the first shift is encouraged to spend time on an informal and formal basis with the family and new resident. There are three assessment periods that must be scheduled:

1. Time where family, the new resident and the staff member are together to assess the new resident's response to new people and the unit.
2. Time where the family are pre-occupied with the family questionnaire (see section on assessment) and the staff member and new resident are left alone. This is an opportunity to assess the new resident's response to being without the family member's support.
3. A time where the staff member and family discuss the family questionnaire and leave the new resident alone. This allows time to assess the response of the new resident to the unit when minimal support is available.

Each of these periods need to be expanded.

One of the easiest ways to provide the new resident familiarity with the staff member assigned and also to decrease some of the anxiety experienced by the family is to sit down to a pre-arranged meal. During the pre-admission meeting, family were asked which food the new resident would enjoy and most likely to eat without much coaxing. That is what is required now.

A common question by staff to such a suggestion is "What if the meal mother will eat is chicken, but chicken is not scheduled for the day of admission?" I have found that many families are willing to make admission as bearable as possible. When they learn the meal may assist in the transition, they are usually willing to bring it from home, or pay to have it delivered from a nearby restaurant. Knowing that such an investment of time or money is important to help mother or father adapt more effectively to the transition is often enough motivation.

I do not dispute that some new admissions will not have family available to provide such a support or at some point family may refuse such a responsibility. It is better to deal with the exceptions as they arise and have the supports in place, rather than to eliminate the supports because there may be exceptions. If family are not given direction on what they can do to help, then it is not known whether they will or not. Commonly, such an active role as providing the first meal is an excellent opportunity for family to decrease much of the guilt that is experienced about putting mother in a long term care facility.

This meal must be in a room that is free from other stimuli – a location where there is a fair bit of certainty that other residents will not be milling around (remember, keep the stimuli to a minimum). That location can be an activity room or a small lounge not in use, or the dining room after everyone else has finished lunch and the room has been vacated.

During the first four hours, an opportunity should be provided for the resident and staff to be alone, and also a time where the resident is left by himself, assessing this person's response to each new situation and event. The goal is to gain as much information as quickly as possible to determine what interventions or strategies will be required by other staff to provide the needed supports to the new admission.

Staff knowing in advance what will occupy the new resident's time and what the person can easily talk about (identified at the pre–admission meeting) is important. Each of these can be employed to enhance rapport with the new resident, decreasing that person's anxiety. More importantly, they become important interventions to deal with the time when the family leave the unit. There is nothing worse than having the new admission watch their family walk through the unit door. Diverting the new resident's attention from the family exiting is important to prevent potential immediate behavioural changes.

c) Tapping the Family

Family members who have cared for this resident prior to admission become the greatest resource in giving staff direction and insight into the new admission's routine. If they have cared for their parent, or had significant contact with him during the progression of the disease, then they have already tested what works and what doesn't regarding approach, activities, etc.

157

Tapping into this information is essential to prevent staff from covering the same ground and repeating the same mistakes family may have already encountered.

It is during admission that family can be asked to complete the Family Questionnaire (presented in chapter eleven on assessment). While family are completing the questionnaire, staff have an opportunity to assess how well the new admission copes with them not present.

d) Contact with Family

The resident's response to being left alone on the unit needs to be tested while family are still available. In this way if the resident is seriously distressed, family are present to assist in calming him. Then staff, with the family's help, can discuss what strategies can be taken when family finally do walk away.

Staff's time alone with family allows the opportunity to clarify the information package provided at the pre–admission meeting. Staff can detail and answer any questions family may have on: their role within the facility; how they can be involved in the care and activities of their parent; communication channels that can be taken if problems are encountered; philosophy of the care and unit; etc. This is needed knowing that family members are usually inundated with information and concerns prior to admission and it will be valuable for staff to review the admission package to clarify misunderstandings.

At the end of the transition period (the first four hours), the staff member assigned to the new admission can now formulate a basic outline of what needs to be done, how to approach this resident, areas of concerns, etc. and provide a specific report to the staff on duty the next shift.

3. Admission – The Orientation Period

The orientation period is the first three days after admission.

a) Staff Assignment

Assigning staff to this resident the first three days must be well planned. The goal in this period is to have the least number of staff involved with this resident as possible and to gain as much specific information as is available. That requires those staff assigned to the new resident on admission day to be scheduled the same shift for the next three days.

For example: The staff member assigned the new admission during the first four hours must be on duty for the next three days. The person assigned this resident the evening and night shifts must also be on duty the next three days. Determining who is assigned the new admission is based solely on the rotation schedule for those days.

Once the assignment is established, a thorough assessment and communication process can be defined. The day staff member who greeted the resident, is required to report personally what she has discovered about this resident to the person assigned on the afternoon shift. That person is then able to maintain some consistency in approach and expectations from the guidelines established by the initial contact.

The afternoon staff member then reports to a specific staff member on the night shift all of the information that has been gained in the last 12 hours (a summary of the 4 hours spent by the day person plus her assessment of the past 8 hours). The night person reports directly to the returning day staff member what has occurred over the past 16 hours since she was last on the unit. This reporting pattern occurs for three days.

The benefits of such consistency for the first three days is obvious. It provides the new resident with a degree of familiarity of staff assigned to perform care. It also provides three staff the opportunity to collaborate the information obtained during each shift. Staff are then able to quickly determine this resident's immediate needs, strengths and limitations and establish a baseline care plan for subsequent staff who will follow. Staff now have the most accurate direction that can be obtained in the shortest period of time.

b) Introduction to the Care Routine

For the first three days after admission and possibly up to the first seven days, it is important that only the basics in care be completed. Staff need to expect that this resident will not respond positively to the first bath, eating in the dining room the first few meals or sleeping the first few nights. Their responsibility to this new resident during that first week of admission is to help this person gain a degree of familiarity with the unit and its staff before feeling any pressure to perform complicated and threatening tasks.

There is no question that there will be exceptions. There are always exceptions to every approach or program established for the mentally impaired. It is possible that family of a new admission have been unable to perform the bath prior to entry to the unit resulting in the new resident having obvious problems with hygiene or odour that must be rectified. Staff have no choice but to initiate a bath possibly on the first day. That bath will create significant distress for the new resident, potentially causing aggressive or wandering behaviour. Once that bath is completed, staff need to take immediate steps to decrease that resident's anxiety before placing any further demands upon him.

Staff flexibility during the Transition Period is the key to successful admission. This resident will probably not undress the first night or two, wandering the halls instead of sleeping. He will then sit when he is tired for short periods in a chair and probably awake more confused, not knowing whether it is day or night. These qualities should not become a point of concern. They are a normal response by the mentally impaired to the changes occurring. Once a degree of familiarity is gained, staff should see a return to a more normal sleeping pattern within a few days.

Likewise the new resident will not be able to handle eating in the dining room the first few meals. Some new residents may require their meals scheduled before or after everyone else, being allowed to eat in the dining room when there is less commotion. For staff to provide such flexibility, they need a microwave oven (a $300 cost) on the unit to allow them to reheat the meal when he is hungry. In fact for some new residents, light frequent meals that can be "eaten on the run" may be the best option.

Finally, staff need to withhold unnecessary activities – bath, assessment, large group involvement, etc. – until it is obvious that this resident is able to respond to the demands placed upon him. Once there is a decline in anxiety from the initial move to the unit and some degree of familiarity is gained, then gradually introducing the resident to the routines of the unit is possible. Staff cannot be so caught up in the routine of getting things done, that they overlook the consequences it creates for the new resident. Flexibility, the willingness to try and then back off if the person obviously is stressed by the task, separates units who are effective with this clientele from those who are not.

c) Involving Family

Asking family to assist with certain activities is a significant asset to the care team. Identifying for family when staff plan to complete a new component of the care routine or postponing a task (i.e. shaving) until family can arrange to visit may decrease for this resident much of the anxiety that can be experienced.

The most traumatic time for the new resident on any unit is usually the first bath. If possible, staff need to schedule the first bath when they are sure they have the time to invest to complete it without being rushed. This allows staff the opportunity to provide the needed supports – first showing the resident the tub room, having him run the water, accompanying the resident back to his/her bedroom to gather his housecoat and return to the tub room to undress and bathe. It is advantageous to have the initial tub bath completed by the staff member who has gained the greatest rapport with this resident. If possible, all efforts should be made to have a family member in attendance to assist with that first bath on the unit. If family have cared for this resident prior to admission they have completed that person's bath many times and would now be a stabilizing influence to help the resident cope. Even if family have never assisted the resident with a tub bath prior to admission, having them on the unit when the bath is completed to assist staff in comforting the resident is a tremendous asset that will contribute to staff's success.

In each of these examples, staff are taking advantage of the first contact with this resident on every aspect of the care routine to determine the appropriate approach or best intervention needed with the least pressure on the resident. The information gained must be shared with other staff in the preliminary care plan. Once the new resident has settled, the initial care plan can then be updated to reflect the resident's needs as they have evolved.

It is always interesting to encounter the responses to the above admission process by some staff and managers. The frequently heard comment is "This all sounds nice, but in reality it cannot be done or there is no time to do it."

With any intervention discussed throughout this text the choice is a simple one – to do it or not do it. It is the difference between adapting the setting to effectively care for this clientele or forcing this individual to adapt to an environment in which he cannot function. An environment that is beyond his ability to cope, creates for him a detrimental setting in which to live.

Time is not the factor here. No matter what is done or not done, time is a constant. We have demonstrated that not providing the supports identified will result in significant and frequent behavioural outbursts and resistance by the new resident. The consequences of inaction (not setting up the needed intervention strategies) can easily be reflected in the wasting of staff time to control an aggressive resident, and the expenditure of the added energy needed to settle other residents on the unit who have been influenced by this resident's response. Each task that is performed without sensitivity to the person's ability only elevates that person's anxiety further, making the simplest of tasks that could be completed in a supportive setting now impossible to do.

Investing the time to develop and adhere to a supportive admission procedure will lessen the negative impact of admission and decrease the behavioural responses to a more tolerable level. The time invested in taking the appropriate steps to establish an effective admission process is then saved in the decreased need to deal with intense reactionary behaviour by the new admission. In either case time will be invested. The difference is to do problem solving or crisis intervention.

I do not like to be involved in crisis intervention with the mentally impaired. The consequences are disastrous for the resident. Such an approach only elevates his anxiety and can create a negative behavioural response for an extended period of time. The impact of the resultant altercations is to upset other residents on the unit, effecting the ability of staff to perform their care and jeopardizing the safety of staff and residents concerned. The choice is yours – Problem Solving or crisis intervention.

SUMMARY

Some are surprised by the emphasis placed on admission. It is a crucial period. It dictates, whether we spend the next few months attempting to establish the environment and care process based on the person's existing strengths and limitations, or waste valuable energy, resources and time to decrease a substantially high anxiety level until we see the "real" person emerge. We will not know who or what we are really dealing with until the transition shock of admission has subsided.

Chapter Nine

Adapting
The Environment

The environment, if adapted effectively, can be a functional mechanism allowing even a severely impaired resident a considerable degree of independence. The goal in arranging the environment is to keep it as simple as possible, leaving as little to memory as necessary. A process of multiple cuing, having a number of mechanisms to reinforce for this person the needed information is the most effective approach. No mentally impaired resident will relate to all or needs all of the options provided. The more cuing that can be employed, the better the chance many residents will relate to at least one, enhancing their ability to function, decreasing the anxiety experienced.

You will discover two overall themes when discussing adaptation of the environment – making the environment "mentally impaired proof" and keeping it "simple/complicated". Making it mentally impaired proof reflects the philosophy of making the behaviour of the mentally impaired tolerable. When a behaviour occurs that is detrimental (disruptive to others or a safety risk issue), the question is not "how do you stop the resident", but "how do you adapt the environment so the resident will not respond in that manner?" Likewise, the concept of keeping it simple/complicated demonstrates that simple tactics are all that are needed to complicate the issue for the mentally impaired, decreasing the disruptive behaviour or eliminating the safety risk that was experienced.

In one facility I was seated in the resident lounge, assessing the unit. A staff member came running up to me, grabbed my arm and haled me out of the chair, down the hall and into a resident's room. She said "You see, this is why you cannot let the mentally impaired wander." What apparently happened was that a level two mentally impaired resident was walking down the hall. She peered into a bedroom where the bed by the door had a pulsating mattress on top. On the floor, at the foot of the bed and in plain view was an air pump, with a light that blinked off and on. The wandering resident saw the light on the pump. She was attracted to it (if the stimuli is too intense some cannot help but respond). She picked up the pump and started walking away with it. Of course it was still connected to the mattress and plugged into the wall. The mattress came with her and the plug was disconnected. As she headed for the door with her bounty, she bumped into a 29 inch TV on coasters sitting against the wall. That moved so she took it with her as well. This staff member wanted to stop the resident's behaviour by restraining her to a chair or locking all bedroom doors to keep this one resident out of those rooms. On the contrary the challenge was how to change the environment so that she could wander but not encounter the same problem.

All the facility had to do was place the pump in a wood box with a lid, which hid the light and then place the box under the bed. It is now mentally impaired proof – out of sight to the mentally impaired is out of mind. As well, they needed to remove the wheels from the TV stand so that it would be too heavy to move.

As we discuss the environment, the challenge to the reader is to determine how to implement the concepts presented. Most long term care facilities find themselves in the situation of adapting existing units to accommodate the increasing number of this type of resident population. Few facilities have the luxury of building new units from scratch. That means that as problems in the environment are encountered, the staff are challenged to determine the most appropriate solutions, knowing that there are no clear and easily presented answers. Interventions with the mentally impaired are most commonly found by implementing strategies on a process of trial and error. You try it, if it works stay with it, if it doesn't, try something else. This again is the main premise for determining any programming direction that involves the mentally impaired.

Here are a number of environmental strategies and interventions that are of value in any setting.

1) Colour Coded Door Frames

Painting only bedroom doors different colours is of little value to mentally impaired residents. Bedroom doors are usually left open during the day and are only visible when one is standing in front of them. Painting the door frames along with the doors is of more value. The door frames can be seen no matter where one is standing in the hall.

Painting the door frames different colours – red, brown, orange, yellow, etc. may be difficult to colour coordinate aesthetically, but can be of a functional benefit to the mentally impaired. [Caution – pastel blues or greens, tend to wash out to yellow or gray for some older people due to normal aging changes of the eye – bright blues and greens may be seen clearly.]

If my door frame is red, it can easily be spotted from anywhere in the hall. There may be more than one red door frame, but the number of doors to choose from has been decreased dramatically. Before you encourage a resident to find his room by looking for the red door frame, you had better determine if he can identify the colour red.

Large sample paint chips (at least 3" x 5" in size) identical to the colours used on the door frames must be available to staff for assessment purposes. Placing the paint chips in a row in front of the resident and asking him to pick the red one will determine his ability to identify that colour. If he cannot recognize red from the paint chips in front of him, he will be unable to pick the red door frame when walking down the hall. If he can identify the colour, it is imperative that all staff direct him to his room by saying "Find the red door frame and you'll find your room."

The resident may end up looking into all of the rooms with a red door frame until he finds his belongings or articles. The amount of stimuli to sort through has been decreased. If there are 10 bedroom doors in the hall and four colours used, only 2 or 3 will be red.

This same concept can be reversed if you have residents wandering into rooms that are used solely by staff (utility room, housekeeper's closet, etc.). To draw the resident only to bedrooms and decrease the amount of wandering into non-resident areas simply paint those doors and door frames the colour of the wall. They will virtually disappear – if the stimulus is not intense enough, it will be missed or misinterpreted. Not only have you pulled these doors from sight, but you have again decreased the number of doors to choose from.

2. Name Bars

If a person cannot find his room by using the colour code, then name bars are of value. The name bars must be 3" by 18". A name bar that is 1" by 3" cannot be seen. Placing the name bar on a contrasting colour plate helps it to stand out – i.e black and white name bar on a red plastic background, same colour as the door frame. The lettering on the name bar must be simple. Fancy script lettering may look nice, but it only results in making it difficult for the mentally impaired to read. Remember, the more complex you make anything, the less chance the mentally impaired will be able to respond to it.

The name that is used on the name plate must be one the person can relate to. One facility had an 82 year old resident whose name bar read "Bucky Buckman". I was challenged by a ministry representative saying that his name bar was disrespectful and it should read Mr. R. Buckman. "Mr. R." means nothing to the mentally impaired. It requires high cognitive ability to be able to interpret letters to mean words. Besides this man had been Bucky Buckman for 82 years of his life, and this is what he related to.

Before you ask a resident to find his room by looking for his name, you had better determine whether he is capable of reading his name. Each unit should have 4 dummy name bars (these can be staff names). Place the 4 dummy name bars and the resident's name bar in front of him and ask him to pick out his name. If he is unable to identify his name from the five in front of him, he will be unable to identify it on the wall outside his door.

Remember to lessen the stimuli. If the person can only relate to his first name, then the name bar on his door frame should only have his first name on it. The more you clutter something for the mentally impaired, the less able they are to identify the usable information.

3. Resident's Picture

Having the resident's picture above or below his name bar may also be of assistance. If there is a concern that the pictures may be easily torn off the wall, Plexiglas covers can be placed over them and bolted to the wall.

Before using the person's picture as a cue to find his room, you had better determine if the resident can recognize himself. A resident who is 84 years old in the picture, but believes he is 42, may not know who he is looking at.

Place five pictures in front of the resident, one of him and one of four others. Then ask him to pick out his picture. If he can't pick it out when it is in front of him, he will be unable to pick it out when it is on the wall outside his room.

There is no need to place a resident's picture on the door frame if that person is unable to identify it and use it to find his room. The only door frames that should have pictures are those door frames of residents who can use them. To have 25 pictures on the wall, each next to the appropriate door frame of the specific resident, when only five residents are able to relate to pictures only clutters the unit and makes it difficult for those five residents to find their picture. To have five doors frames with pictures eliminates for those residents the amount of information that must be sorted. The goal is to simplify the unit.

4. Identifying Decor

For those residents who cannot relate to the coloured door frames, name bars or picture, then a forth option may be available. Having a decoration on the bedroom door that is not duplicated on any other door is of help to some. The decoration needs to be something very specific to this resident so that he can relate to it, usually an object or picture of something in his/her past. A bell on the door of a resident whose name was Mrs. Bell, a bank poster on the door of a resident who was an ex–bank manager, etc.

The need for such cuing was emphasized by a mentally impaired resident of one facility (often the major source for many of the interventions discovered). This gentleman found a magic marker. He then proceeded to make "X" markings from the lounge to the door of his room. With those markings, he was able to find his room. He created for himself a trail to follow.

What I admired about that unit is they left the markings on the wall for as long as he could use them. They knew that if he needed them, they were important. They fought off many demands to paint that wall by those who did not understand its

168

importance. Their commitment to the philosophy they professed – Quality of Life for their residents, outweighed any need to aesthetically improve the looks of that wall.

By the way, none of the environmental cues mentioned above work for every mentally impaired resident who is unable to find his room. Usually 10% who cannot find their room will be able to relate to the coloured door frames, another 10% to the name bar, another 10% to their picture and another 10% to the individualized decor. How does that help? It is simple. If you have ten residents who cannot find their room, by implementing the cuing, you now only have six residents who cannot find their room. I'd rather have six than ten. We have not solved the problem, but made it more tolerable, the basic philosophy for any intervention implemented.

PERSONALIZING THE ROOM

Whatever assists the person in finding his room (colour, name bar, picture, decor) can also be used to assist the resident to identify his bed (important in a semi–private or ward room). If a cuing device works in one setting, the goal is to use it for other settings as well. Placing the name bar, colour plate, picture or decoration on the foot board of the bed may decrease the amount of rummaging by some residents.

A bulletin board at the head of the bed and to the side is of further help. It is the ideal location for family pictures, greeting or birthday cards, etc. Seeing these articles assists some in knowing they are in the right room, at the right bed.

A personal bedspread brought from home (previously described as an anchor – using one object to identify where you are) helps some mentally impaired to find their room. For those resident's who have not brought a bedspread from home, ask a major retail outlet to bring in a number of bedspreads with different colours and patterns into the facility. Place the spreads in the lounge or auditorium, then allow a few of the mentally impaired residents at a time to scan the spreads until they pick one (remember not all will be able to pick one). Those who are able to pick a specific spread are usually able to do so because the colour or pattern stands out for that person (the stimuli is intense). That spread can now be purchased through the resident's trust account and placed on his bed. It may now become a significant aid to help that person find his room. Remember that even though some residents are able to pick out a specific spread in one location once, it does not mean that all will be able to pick out the same spread when it is placed on their bed. You will not know his ability to use the spread as an anchor until you try it (a process of trial and error).

CALENDARS AND CLOCKS

As mentioned earlier, a clock to some mentally impaired residents is meaningless. A large clock in the room at eye level may be of value to some, but before staff encourage it to be used, the ability of the resident to use it must be assessed (as discussed in chapter twelve). An old fashioned pendulum chime clock located in the lounge may be the most valuable time piece. It is not intended to help residents to know the time, but rather to hook old memory. It is interesting to see the response of some residents when they hear the chimes.

Knowing the day of the week is of little importance to a mentally impaired resident – if I forget it is my bath day, you will remind me. Placing a large bank calendar on the bulletin board in the resident's room is not for the resident, but more for his family and the staff.

If my family visited at 1400 hours and left at 1445 hours, would the afternoon staff be told at report that they were just in? Probably not. Not unless the visit was unusual in some way. If at 1600 hours I say to one of the afternoon staff, "My family doesn't visit me", what is their response? Not knowing my family was just in, their only response can be "They will be in soon!" That is not reality reinforcement. They were just in less then 2 hours before, but the staff member is unable to reinforce it.

The purpose of the calendar is for family to record their visits. If my daughter Kimberly visited at 1400 hours, she is encouraged to write on the calendar the time she was in, how long she stayed and what she discussed or did. If she knows when she plans to visit next, she is encouraged to record that time on the calendar.

Now, when I say to the staff "My family never visits", they need only to take me to the calendar and show me when she was last in, how many times she has been in the last few weeks and when she plans to visit me again. The information may be lost as soon as it is given to the resident, but at least staff are equipped with an appropriate response specific to that person.

Having family record their visits is also an effective assessment tool. On admission, one of the questions asked of family is "How often do you plan to visit?" If they expect to visit every second day, but the calendar shows that they have only been in twice in the last two weeks, then staff have an opportunity to intervene on a potential problem. Without the calendar, it would be difficult to know that a possible problem exists until it is well advanced and possibly too difficult to resolve.

The calendar can communicate to staff very important personal information as well – birthdays (self and family members), anniversaries, etc. This way staff can talk with any resident about those events while performing care, reinforcing the event as well as the passage of time.

LOCATOR SIGNS

What is in my closet or bedside table? If the only way to know is by memory, then the mentally impaired are lost.

Locator signs can assist some mentally impaired residents to find things in their room. Placing a sign on the door of my closet, dresser or bedside table that has the word describing the article and a picture of it may be all that is needed. A large sign on my closet door with the words and pictures indicating shirts, pants, shoes and a sign showing a pipe, hair brush, etc. for the door at my bedside table compensates for my memory loss. Before using any signs, it is again important to assess the resident's ability to read and understand either the pictures or the words.

Locator signs on washroom doors, whether the door is accessed from within the resident's room or from the hall, are necessary. The sign must be bright, contrasting against the colour of the door, large, with the word "washroom" and a picture of a toilet. Even though the washroom may be attached to a resident's room, if the door is closed, the person will not find it, wandering in the hall looking for the toilet and the delay may result in incontinence. Leave nothing to memory. If the resident cannot see it, he cannot find it.

MIRRORS

Most of us have an "internal picture" of ourselves. This can be demonstrated simply enough. How many times has someone taken a snapshot of you and you exclaimed – "That's not me. I don't look like that." That snapshot is in conflict with your own internal picture, how you believe you look.

At this moment what can you see of yourself?

Your hands, the rest of your body, but you cannot see your face. The only time you have an opportunity to see your face is when you look in the mirror.

The same is true with a mentally impaired resident. If I am mentally impaired, I cannot see my face. I am virtually looking from the inside out. All I see are my hands and body. If, in my mind's eye I see myself as 42, but in actual fact I am 85, there is nothing to contradict my belief.

Like everything else discussed, mirrors are of value for some mentally impaired, or create agitation in others and elicit peculiar responses in still others.

A mirror can cause agitated behaviour in some mentally impaired. If a mentally impaired resident has the ability to know that he is looking at his reflection in a mirror, he will experience considerable difficulty. Due to his memory loss, he sees himself in his mind as 42 years old, but in actual fact he is 84. Looking at his reflection he will experience a state called Reality Shock. This is a situation where the person is suddenly confronted with something that contrasts with his beliefs. When this resident sees his reflection in the mirror and he <u>knows</u> it is him, the contradiction creates intense and immediate confusion. His anxiety level then increases to a panic state, he becomes agitated and may break the mirror. For this individual, a mirror must not be in his room and the value of placing him in front of a mirror must be greater than the consequences created when he sees himself.

Other mentally impaired residents do not have the cognitive ability to know that what they are seeing when they look in a mirror is their own reflection. The mirror in that situation then initiates a very different behavioural response. This resident will talk to their reflection, believing it is someone else. The stimulus for this person is too obscure, easily causing him to misinterpret what he sees. In fact the mirror may result in an 82 year old resident telling you that he just saw his father where in actual fact he was looking at himself. There is no question that the location of a mirror for this resident is of significant importance. If a mirror is located in this resident's room where he can see it while lying in bed, then staff may find him very restless or unable to sleep at night. It would be rude to sleep when you have a visitor or frightening if you believed there was someone else in the room that you did not know.

The location of a mirror on any unit must be considered carefully. In one facility a full length mirror was at the end of the hall. It was interesting to watch certain mentally impaired residents walk down the hall. As they caught sight of themselves in the mirror, they stepped to the other side of the hall, and then moved back again. Obviously they were trying to get out of the way of the person coming towards them (seeing their own reflection in the mirror). A mirror in this location can contribute to some residents falling or becoming aggressive, getting angry when they cannot get out of the way of the other person.

Another facility had a mirror located between two windows in every resident bedroom. I asked a staff member to look through the window and describe what she saw – "snow on the ground". I asked her to look through the mirror next to the window, or better yet through what looks like the middle window, and describe what she saw – she said "herself." My response in return was "You had better let that person in, she will get cold out there in the snow." This is the possible perception of a level two mentally impaired resident. Instead of seeing a mirror and two windows, a mentally impaired resident may see three windows – snow on either side and a person in the middle one – an obscure stimulus that may cause considerable anxiety and inappropriate behaviour.

Glass covering pictures or paintings on the hallway walls may cause a similar response as mirrors. Non–glare glass should be used. If not, the picture will be lost and the mentally impaired resident will talk to his reflection.

The way that mentally impaired residents view and respond to mirrors solidifies well the concepts of Supportive Therapy. When one focuses on the strengths of the mentally impaired rather than their limitations you cannot help but be impressed by their ability to take the little information available to them and use the few remaining analytical skills to be able to make sense of what they see. It emphasizes well the importance of our understanding the world as they see it in order to assist them to function.

HOOKING OLD MEMORY

If the lounge looks like a waiting room, I will wait for only so long and if nothing happens I will leave. If the dining room is just a large room with a number of tables in it, then you may have a problem with my sitting there to eat. Being unable to remember that I am living in a long term care facility makes it difficult to relate to either the lounge or the dining room if they do not look like anything familiar from my past.

The dining room must look like a dining room and the lounge look like a living room. You do not have to tell me what to do when I see a sofa, I sit. You do not have to tell me where to eat when I see the proper table. In renovating units, the instructions given to staff are simple – make this room your dining room or living room in your home. How would you decorate it?

If you "hook" old memory, the chances are great that a mentally impaired resident may respond appropriately to what he/she is seeing. Furniture is now available that is attractive and home–like in appearance, but easy to maintain and treated against incontinence. Using end tables, table lamps and floor lamps adds the needed touch. There is always the concern that lamps can be knocked over, so you adapt the environment to suite the residents – bolt the table lamps to the table from the bottom (similar to what is done in motel rooms), bolt the floor lamps to the floor. The more the room can look normal, the more the behaviour that will be elicited will be normal.

Plants, pictures, books, book shelves are all essential in any living environment. Pictures on the walls need only be secured by screwing them to the wall so that they are not easily knocked down. Some staff are afraid that mentally impaired residents may eat the plants (a behaviour I have rarely encountered). Just adapt the environment – have only eatable plants or at least those that are not dangerous if taken internally.

A display case made of break–proof glass located in the lounge can contain articles of historic significance and become quite a conversation piece for the residents. Changing the articles every few months keeps the case interesting. A local museum, the facility's volunteers, or auxiliary, can be encouraged to provide the different articles needed.

MULTIPLE LOUNGES/ALTERNATE DINING ROOMS

An appropriate living environment for the mentally impaired must be one that limits the amount of stimuli that can be encountered. One large lounge with 30 or more residents is too much activity for many mentally impaired, especially if that lounge is also where the radio and TV are located.

It is important to separate those residents who can easily agitate others from those who are sensitive to such stimuli. Multiple small lounges allow residents to be placed in a room that best suits them. Usually three smaller lounges are best, a TV room, a music room and a quiet room providing staff the needed flexibility in locating residents based on their functioning ability and sensitivity to stimuli.

For some residents, having a comfortable chair and a TV or radio in their room may be a viable option, allowing staff the opportunity to provide certain residents periods alone in a quiet environment.

The dining room must be versatile. Residents who are able to feed themselves, but are easily distracted, require little to take their attention from their meal. A small dining room for those who need to be fed or can be disruptive, allows the high functioning mentally impaired to concentrate on their meal without being distracted.

PARKS

An outside enclosed park is an asset to any unit. A park enclosed by a chain linked fence will often not be sufficient. Certain wanderers may leave an enclosed area, not from the desire to leave the building or property, but only from being attracted to what they see on the other side of the fence – children playing, or a garden that needs tending in the next yard. A chain linked fence allows the mentally impaired resident to see what is on the other side, resulting in some scaling over the top and leaving the courtyard.

The best enclosure is one that appears as a solid wall to the mentally impaired, such as hedging in front of a louvered wooden fence. Even though one can see through the fence at a certain angle, to the mentally impaired the wall appears solid, decreasing the tendency to go over the wall to the next yard.

The walking path in the park needs to be a winding walkway that starts and ends at the door to the unit. When the resident walks the path, he is virtually led away and back to the unit – he will wander the unit, go out the door, wander in the park and return to wander the unit, a never ending loop.

The ideal park is one that is landscaped with bushes, a gazebo and benches strategically placed so the wanderer has resting points. These resting stations need something to attract him to stop, such as raised gardens or flower beds which bring the plants into view and allow the resident to till the soil or touch the flowers or pick them without stooping. Bird feeders add a nice touch.

I have seen some very attractive and functional enclosed courtyards for the mentally impaired that are rarely used. On any unit, the mentally impaired are often told directly or indirectly (by security devices), not to go out any doors. Yet they are being told (during nice weather only) to go out the door that leads to the courtyard. The residents do not have the cognitive ability to function under such confusing and contradictory instructions.

The only way that the mentally impaired will utilize a courtyard is if they are drawn out. Placing an automatic opening patio door in the wandering path is one answer. As the wanderer crosses the sensor to the patio door, it opens. The person will then be attracted through it (looking for something familiar) and will walk the leading pathway (starts and ends at the patio door) through the courtyard. On returning to the door, the sensor will be activated again, the patio door will open and the person will enter the unit. The process is repeated continually. In this way the unit has created an effective wandering loop. By the way, if the weather is poor, just flip the switch to the patio door, shutting off the sensor. The resident will walk up to the door, nothing happens, he will then move down the hall.

P.A. SYSTEM, TELEVISION AND RADIO

You are a mentally impaired resident

Living in a long term care facility/
You are sitting alone in the lounge/
Suddenly there is a voice from nowhere/

What is your response?

As soon as the P.A. speaker sounds off with a message, some mentally impaired residents begin talking aloud. It takes a great deal of cognitive ability to know the voice is coming from a speaker, connected by wire to the front office.

Even cognitively well residents in most facilities do not relate to random P.A. announcements. How often do activity staff go to the unit to get residents for an activity even though the announcement was just made? By the time a cognitively well resident is aware that the message concerns him and he is attentive, the message is over. This even happens to staff. How often has someone come to you and said "That page was for you, didn't you hear it?"

To decrease the stimuli on a unit, staff must eliminate unnecessary noise. The most appropriate use of the P.A. is to establish a specific time each morning for all resident announcements. Having announcements each morning between 0900 and 0910 hours encourages the cognitively well residents to be more attentive, rather than having to listen to the barrage of random messages bombarding them each day. The goal is to eliminate the use of the P.A. systems. Supplying key personnel with a beeper, (maintenance staff, administrator, director of nursing) and restricting the P.A. to emergency calls only, which makes the environment a much quieter and more comfortable setting for all concerned.

Many mentally impaired residents are incapable of watching TV, for the simple reason that it moves too fast from one scene to another − at one moment you are watching a soap commercial and the next you see a car blow up. Those mentally impaired who do watch TV, probably do so from old behaviour and old memory. Ask a male, mentally impaired resident, watching a hockey game, who is playing and what is the score of a game on TV, and he will be unable to tell you. If he is able to sit for extended periods in front of the TV during a hockey game, it is likely old behaviour for him. He has watched hockey games all of his life and the behaviour is familiar to him. Similarly, another resident may be watching a soap opera and know nothing of what is happening or who is involved. Again it may only be old behaviour.

One thing that I will consciously do when touring a unit is to go straight to the lounge and turn off the TV. Once off, I will stand there for a moment to see if there is any response at all from the residents sitting in that lounge, either a comment "I was watching that" or some movement to show that a person is distressed by it being off. More often than not there is no response, only an immediate quieting of the lounge. Unfortunately, turning on the TV becomes an immediate habit of some staff. As soon as they walk into the lounge, the TV is switched on and left on all day. If the goal is to decrease the amount of stimuli on the unit, staff must be consciously aware of that at all times. There are certain noises and disruptions that cannot be avoided on a unit of 30 residents. Those that can be controlled must be eliminated.

If the TV in the lounge is located on the floor, you may find your wandering residents are always attracted to it. The wanderer is often drawn to the greatest stimuli. Frequently this resident walks to the TV, stands in front of it, strokes it, turns the dials, etc. This sets the stage for a potential scenario for an aggressive outburst from those watching the program (on a mixed unit which includes cognitively well residents). To solve the problem, the TV need only be attached to the wall at above eye level and tilted slightly forward. This keeps the TV out of view from the wanderer, making him less likely to disrupt others watching it.

Placing the TV at such a height then becomes an inconvenience for those who want to choose the channel and control the volume. What is needed is a remote controlled TV, where the remote control is secured to a table top where the cognitively well residents sit. This allows them to be independent while watching TV, and the remote control is too small for the mentally impaired to be attracted to it.

If, for proper viewing, the TV needs to be placed at a distance from those watching it, requiring the volume to be turned high to hear it, creating more noise. Maintenance can easily install external speakers to the TV. These speakers can be located at the back of the lounge allowing those residents who are watching a program to hear it and still keep the volume low. If a cognitively well resident has a hearing problem and needs the volume higher than anyone else, attaching volume controlled earphones to the speakers allows this resident to hear the program without disturbing others.

When I find the radio in the resident's lounge at a station playing music I believe residents cannot relate to, I will turn the channel without asking. The tempo, the accentuated down beat and the unintelligible lyrics of modern music has the potential of agitating the mentally impaired (let alone parents). Soothing conventional music is more relaxing, having the opposite effect. In fact, you know if you have the right music coming from the radio when many of your young staff complain that they do not like the station that is playing.

As with everything else we have discussed, music to some mentally impaired is noise to others. Constant music piped in over the P.A. system can create sensory overload for the mentally impaired or anyone else for that matter. Why is it that during a meeting in the board room, staff or managers want the P.A. turned off? To demonstrate the impact of such constant stimuli, leave the piped in music on during your next meeting and see how difficult it is for all to concentrate on what is being said. This exercise usually results in the music being turned off in the halls. The goal in the environment of the mentally impaired is to decrease stimuli.

Fire drills can create the most havoc with the mentally impaired. Of course there is no value to warn staff in advance of a pending fire drill, but it is necessary to be prepared for its effects. The anxiety level of the mentally impaired is increased dramatically during the drill. The ability of any resident to immediately respond to any further stress afterwards is severely restricted. Trying to bath a mentally impaired resident who has just gone through a fire drill that he does not understand is impossible. Trying to run a scheduled activity program with a group of mentally impaired residents just after a fire drill is useless. The mentally impaired must be allowed to settle before the routine of the unit is resumed. Whoever is pulling the fire alarm must know that for at least one to two hours afterwards, activities involving mentally impaired residents are cancelled or postponed until "things return to normal".

STAFF IDENTIFICATION

Staff name tags are necessary and commonly used. Name tags that are small, with small printing, containing too much information or have a shiny surface (brass or gold), are of little value. Name tags need to be large with the staff member's first name only. There is no need for the department to be identified on the name tag, those words have little meaning to many of the mentally impaired. Colour coding name tags to identify departments may have a better impact – red for housekeeping, blue for nursing, etc.

There has been some controversy over staff wearing uniforms or street clothes during work. The white uniform is not necessary, but some consistency in dress is important. If a resident has difficulty identifying staff from other residents, how does he know who is taking him to the bathroom, if that person is wearing the same clothes as the people who live there? If uniforms are not worn, then colour coding identifying departments is the other option – nursing will wear a white/blue combination, white top/blue pants, visa versa; housekeeping will wear green, dietary yellow, etc.

SUMMARY

Working with the mentally impaired requires an investment of energy into new and innovative techniques and approaches. We are forging a new philosophy in what we do and how we do it. Our success can be measured by the response of the residents within our care.

It is one thing to provide options in how to care for the mentally impaired effectively, it is another to decide which of those options is the most appropriate with any one resident. In order to be as supportive as possible, we must be able to effectively determine our direction in care with each resident we encounter.

Chapter Ten

Care Analysis

The mentally impaired elderly are a highly complex clientele. Yet there is still the tendency of some staff to limit their expectations of a resident's behaviour to a "black/white" or "this/that" rationale – simple answers to describe a very complex problem.

Imagine:

You are an 84 year old
Mentally impaired resident
You have been a chronic chain smoker most of your life/
Staff of the facility decide your smoking should be limited
To one cigarette an hour/

You want a cigarette/
You find a staff member
Walk up to that person and say
"Cigarette, cigarette, cigarette, cigarette,..." continuously/

Staff do not give in/
They hold you to one cigarette an hour/
Whenever you approach the desk
Calling for a cigarette
Staff take you to your room/

If you are sitting quietly in your room/
No one dares talk to you
Fearing you will start the behaviour again/
If they see you walking down the hall towards them
They duck into a bedroom until you go by
To avoid having you ask for a cigarette/

After about 9 months
Staff finally gave in/

Giving you a cigarette whenever you want it/

Would that stop your behaviour?

This is an actual case. The resident's behaviour and staff's response occurred as described. At the ninth month the staff's frustration in restricting this lady to one cigarette an hour reached its limit. They decided the program was not worth the effort and now gave her a cigarette whenever she wanted one hoping that would stop her behaviour. Nothing changed. Staff soon found that even though she just finished a cigarette, she would approach them demanding another. They concluded that her actions were intentional in order to gain attention.

There could be nothing further from the truth. This resident's cognitive ability was very limited, she did not know where she was nor who the people were around her. Her behaviour was influenced by a number of factors that went far beyond the simple request for a cigarette. One of the major motivators for her actions was uncovered in a conversation with her family well after the final actions taken by staff (shared later in this discussion). The family stated that their mother always had a cigarette in her hand or in the ash tray, she was a chronic chain smoker for years. What staff experienced now was simply "old behaviour".

This lady now has inadvertently become conditioned − to see someone is to elicit from her the request for a cigarette (similar to conditioning an animal to salivate when it hears a bell). Little cognitive ability was required, yet staff believed that she intentionally knew what she was doing because she knew to go to the nursing station. That assessment was inaccurate as well. Her attraction to the nursing station was simple. It was the only place on the unit where anyone would stand in one place for an extended period of time. As soon as someone went behind the desk, whether it was the doctor, nurse, housekeeper or manager, she would approach with her call "Cigarette, cigarette, . . ." She knew that cigarettes were to be found in that location, but what the location was had no meaning for this resident. This is no different than another mentally impaired resident going to the bathroom to urinate or to the dining room to eat, but not knowing what those rooms were or what they were called.

Lastly, staff continually emphasized that "she just had a cigarette", believing that she was aware of that, therefore her asking again meant that she just wanted attention. Again staff had not looked closely enough at this resident's situation. This lady had very poor memory retention. The staff were aware of her just finishing a cigarette, she wasn't. She forgot about a cigarette just as soon as she put it out, requesting another as though she hadn't had one. In this case, staff did not have a formal mechanism to analyze her behaviour and understand the rationale behind her actions.

The staff finally decided after nine months of unsuccessfully "battling" to give this resident a cigarette whenever she wanted one. Unfortunately that intervention was not well planned or consistent. Without direction on how staff were to ensure that she would receive a cigarette as often as she wanted, it meant that she could receive one only when nursing staff were free, which was infrequent at best. Furthermore, some staff still avoided this lady rather than give her a cigarette believing that she was in control of her behaviour and they didn't want to "give in". The result was that the resident's behaviour continued with the same intensity as before. When giving her cigarettes "freely" didn't work the staff decided their only recourse was to sedate her. That didn't stop her from approaching the desk, so they now restrained her.

As an outsider to this situation you can be as critical as you want about the staff's interventions. Work with this resident every day for nine months, encountering this behaviour repeatedly every shift and then tell me how objective you will be. Sometimes when you are too close to the problem, it is "too hard to see the forest for the trees", making it difficult to be objective when resolving it. If staff are not given a concrete, objective mechanism to analyze a situation, then their interventions will always be inappropriate or ineffective.

Once staff in this case were required to analyze this lady's behaviour through a process called Care Analysis, they had a better understanding of why it was occurring. Looking deeper into the causative factors uncovered three possible reasons for her actions: "old memory" or previous lifestyle, conditioning and memory loss. With these facts at hand, staff were now able to identify what was needed and how best to accomplish it.

In this case it was important to ask staff why they felt this lady's smoking should be restricted in the first place. The staff's response was a concern about safety, a legitimate problem.

183

Unfortunately, they believed that limiting her smoking would eliminate that concern. Instead it created a more difficult problem.

Staff needed to focus on their concern, not on her smoking. A major focus of Supportive Therapy is that you cannot stop the behaviour of the mentally impaired, you can only make it tolerable. The guideline of one cigarette an hour should have represented the minimum number of cigarettes given, not the maximum. That meant that she could smoke as much as she wanted as long as she was supervised. The interventions that were required to ensure safety were as follows:

- the resident was properly fitted with a smoking apron that looked like a normal apron covering her chest and lap when she sat
- the ash tray provided to her was to be large and deep, to prevent her cigarettes from rolling out and to ensure the ashes ended up in the ash tray
- all staff (including nurse, housekeeping, recreation, maintenance, management, etc.) were encouraged to give her a cigarette whenever they were in the lounge
- cognitively well residents were asked to supervise her smoking when they sat in the lounge near her
- volunteers were assigned to supervise her smoking whenever they were free
- staff who smoked were allowed to sit and have a cigarette with her when they were free (that freedom would raise a few eyebrows in some facilities)
- staff were encouraged to employ diversional activity (involvement in specific tasks) when no one was available to supervise her smoking

If she could not afford the number of cigarettes that she was smoking, then local community groups (Kiwanas, Kinsmen, etc.), the auxiliary or volunteers of the facility were encouraged to donate a cash fund to the unit. This allowed the unit to have extra cigarettes on hand for those who ran out.

Staff now had available to them a realistic intervention strategy that enhanced their ability to cope with the repetitive behaviour. More importantly they realized their limitations in stopping the behaviour, given this lady's past history and memory loss.

What is most important about this discussion is the process – before staff could define their direction of care, they had to thoroughly analyze the residents behaviour.

It is necessary to identify another example that demonstrates the need for effective analysis. Let us discuss a resident we will call Marg. The unit where Marg lived was very structured in its routine and programs. Supper was at 1630 hours and residents were prepared for bed at 1700 hours, even though they were not put to bed at that time.

Marg's history of fighting staff resulted in her being labeled aggressive. Staff decided it was best to prepare Marg for bed first for two reasons. One reason was that her room was the first one down the hall (that rationale must have made sense to someone). The other reason was that staff knew she would be aggressive during the procedure and felt they may as well fight the "13 rounds" with her now as opposed to later.

The aggressive label attached to Marg resulted in staff not warning her in advance that they were going to undress her and prepare her for bed. They felt if they told her what they were going to do, she would become aggressive even before they started. Their strategy was to have two staff wait inside the bathroom by the door (the door opened into the hallway). One staff member stood inside the door on one side, another on the other side and they waited.

Marg was a wanderer. As soon as Marg reached the bathroom door, they closed their trap – they whisked her into the washroom, undressed her, put her nightgown on her and returned her to the hall. When released into the hall, Marg wandered about the unit pounding her fist and yelling "They're stealing my clothes, they're stealing my clothes . . ." from 5 PM until midnight. It was not surprising that the only way staff could get her to settle was to repeat her sedation (sleeping pill) at 11 PM.

To the staff this was just Marg, always aggressive no matter what you did with her! They believed they were justified in their tactics because they had no other choice – a black/white, this/that rationale to a complex problem. A situation like this is gradual in its development, but common in its course. It is difficult to be objective when you are confronted with the same problem day after day. The staff could not see that their approach mattered when it came to Marg.

No matter what resident behaviour we discuss, it is difficult to determine what is causing it. There is no staff member that can know any one resident totally. It requires the combined efforts of the entire team to paint the picture of who this person is and what is happening.

The care conference is the focal point for that sharing. A way to make the conference a highly valuable problem solving opportunity is by using a technique called Care Analysis – a process of defining the causative factors to any identified care issue. Care Analysis is a problem identification mechanism. It allows all members of the team to brainstorm what may be causing a resident's behaviour or change in functioning.

Care Analysis is a formal mechanism that is utilized during the team conference. At the care conference, a flip chart is placed in front of the group and a staff member is asked to become the recorder. The recorder's job is to first write on the flip chart a concern or behaviour (called a care issue) that staff are having difficulty with regarding a specific resident (i.e. wandering, aggression, hoarding, etc.). All staff are then asked to give all the possible reasons why any resident who is mentally impaired may perform in that manner. Once all the reasons are identified, then staff are asked which on the list they believe applies to this resident. That becomes the Nursing Diagnosis on the resident care plan. Probably the best way to demonstrate this process is to discuss Marg and her aggressive behaviour.

AGGRESSIVE BEHAVIOUR

In Marg's case the care issue written on the top of the flip chart was as follows:

Aggressive when asked to perform care tasks.

Marg became aggressive during toileting, dressing, etc., whether she was asked in advance or whether the task was just done.

Imagine that you know Marg and are part of the care conference. Place Marg aside in your mind for a moment and identify all the possible reasons why any mentally impaired resident may become aggressive when asked to perform care tasks. That list would probably include the following:

Need for Privacy
Control
Comprehension (language & instructions)
Pressuring
Past Experience
Approach
Need to Perform
Environment
Lifestyle
Medication
Timing
Fear
Progressive Agitation
Old Behaviour
Bombarding
False Cuing
Personality Conflict
Values
Disease

It is important at this time to expand on each of these issues to demonstrate again the vulnerability of the individual we are discussing and detail the perceptions and responses of the mentally impaired.

1. Need for Privacy

Just because a person is mentally impaired does not mean that he/she is not aware of being exposed. On one unit staff experienced considerable resistive and aggressive behaviour when toileting female residents. The washroom normally used was a large communal washroom with 4 toilets and 4 sinks. Toileting involved at least four residents or more and two or three staff at a time in that one location.

After some discussion with staff, they decided to use a staff washroom down the hall for those residents who were the hardest to handle. That washroom contained one sink and one toilet and had a door that could be closed. Aggressive outbursts during toileting decreased to almost nil from that point on, due to the simple fact that the female residents were provided the needed privacy.

2. Control

I have walked onto units and met individuals that seemed to be in complete control, dressed properly and presenting themselves just "so". When I asked staff if that person was a volunteer, they usually told me the person I met was one of the most confused residents living on the unit.

The need to demonstrate one is in control may still be present even though the person is mentally impaired. This perception stems from the fact that some level two residents do not believe they are sick. Instead they may believe they are a volunteer or visitor on the unit.

One lady in her 70's was an ex–school teacher and was now very impaired mentally. She was always dressed immaculately and walked about the unit believing she was there to help others. While conducting an assessment on her, she stopped me abruptly within minutes of my beginning our conversation and said "You are asking me questions aren't you? Well, I won't answer any more of your questions." She refused to talk with me from that point on. This lady dealt with her increasing anxiety when she was incapable of functioning by avoiding situations where she felt pressured. If she could not leave those situations, she would then become aggressive. Try toileting a resident who believes she can toilet herself, but who couldn't do it by herself if her life depended on it. When not allowed to avoid the task, such a resident would feel pressured, responding to the stress by becoming aggressive.

Mentally impaired residents who believe they are still in control may become aggressive during care – dressing, toileting etc. – simply from the fact they do not believe they need any help, even though they are totally incapable of performing effectively on their own.

3. Comprehension (Language & Task)

Abstract terms and directions to some mentally impaired residents have little meaning. The words "Go to the dining room" may be too complex to comprehend. The instructions may need to be simplified to be understood – "I want you to go and sit at the table where you eat and have your lunch." In actual fact, that is what "go to the dining room" means. The inability to understand what a person is saying increases frustration and anxiety resulting in an aggressive response.

Furthermore, the resident's loss of ability to identify objects may result in his being unable to understand the simplest requests being asked – "I want you to sit on the toilet." Not being able to identify what a toilet is can create considerable anxiety. If the word has no meaning, then what is being asked is not understood.

The ability of a resident to remember the sequence of a task may also be lost. To follow instructions, one must be able to remember them. Some mentally impaired residents can remember the first thing asked, but moving to the second step results in forgetting the first was completed, losing track of the third, and so on. The resident becomes so confused, that his frustration level increases, causing an agitated response. To some mentally impaired residents, each task is a series of problems. If cognition or problem solving ability is impaired, the simplest task becomes very complex.

4. Pressuring

The time provided by staff and the time needed by the resident to complete a task may not be the same. The resident simply cannot undress or wash himself in the time allotted. He is physically or cognitively unable to move fast enough through the task in order to complete it. This results in the feeling of being pressured, causing an agitated response.

5. Past Experience

We do not always know what some of our residents have encountered while living in our facility or under the care of others prior to their contact with us. Physical or mental abuse of the mentally impaired is always a possibility (abuse is discussed later in this chapter). Such an experience of being abused may now initiate a defensive reaction during certain tasks.

6. Approach

We have discussed repeatedly how an inappropriate approach will elicit an aggressive response. Staff who are very structured in their care routine often encounter an aggressive response from the mentally impaired due to their lack of flexibility. Staff who are more supportive, providing time and being aware of the individual's limits will encounter little aggressive behaviour.

7. Need to Perform

Some mentally impaired residents are aware of what they want to do but just cannot do it. They have lost hand–eye movement, the ability to control coordinated movements (apraxia) even though they cognitively know how to complete a task. I may know how to button my shirt and what a buttoned shirt looks like, my problem is that I cannot manipulate my fingers. The frustration level in this situation becomes unbearable, resulting in an aggressive response.

8. Environment

Where you want me to undress or bathe is too cold or too hot, too large or too small, too noisy or too quiet, too light or too dark, etc. Any extreme in any one of these areas may create for one mentally impaired or another some difficulty. This results in the person just not wanting to do what you are asking in that location. He becomes aggressive as a result.

9. Lifestyle

Some people have their shower or bath in the morning – to wake up. Others have their shower or bath in the evening – to help them sleep. I have never used an electric razor, only a straight razor. What you want me to do is not my normal way of doing things. To prevent you from doing something that is not natural to me, I become aggressive.

10. Medications

The medications that can cause aggressive outbursts are the same ones that are used to prevent it – sedatives. A sedative generally works by decreasing an individual's energy level, decreasing the ability or desire to become aggressive. That effect also decreases the person's energy level in performing almost anything else. The resident who is sedated and asked to perform certain tasks feels pressured to exert himself when he has little desire or ability to do so. That pressuring can result in a resistive response and a burst of aggressive behaviour.

11. Timing

For some mentally impaired it is best to do certain aspects of their care first thing in the morning when they are well rested, than to perform that same care in the evening when they are tired. When they are tired, they have little patience and feel pressured. However the opposite is also true (like everything else involving the mentally impaired). It may be best to perform certain care tasks with some mentally impaired residents in the evening when they are tired, than in the morning when they are rested. In the morning, they have too much energy and they will fight you, whereas in the evening when they are tired they are less resistive.

12. Fear

If I am experiencing a great deal of anxiety, one thing I do not want is to be placed in a further anxiety provoking situation.

The mentally impaired have a significant fear of the unknown. Things that they cannot relate to will only cause a further elevation of their anxiety to an eventual panic state. Probably the best example that demonstrates this is when staff placed an 82 year old, level two mentally impaired resident in a whirlpool tub using a lift. He probably never saw such devices even when he was cognitively well, making the equipment foreign to him. His being asked to get into a tub of swirling water only results in him fighting staff. Place that same person in a normal tub, and he may be less aggressive.

A resident's fear can also be intensified by other situations as well.

Imagine:

I am a mentally impaired male resident
Over six foot tall
I weigh 240 pounds/
It is very hard for me
To get out of my chair/

I am approached by a nurse

191

Who is five and a half feet tall /
She weighs 115 pounds/
She is going to lift me out of my chair/

That nurse is probably very skilled and knows the necessary body mechanics that will allow her to successfully assist such a large resident from his chair. The problem does not lie with the staff member, it is with the mentally impaired male resident who does not know her, nor her skills. All he sees is a small, young woman trying to pick him up. His fear is that she will drop him, so he fights or resists her. Have another staff member who is taller and heavier do the same task and he will probably be less resistive.

There are many examples that demonstrate how our setting can intensify the fear of the mentally impaired.

Having two staff help a naked, level two mentally impaired resident into a tub, requiring him to lift his leg over the edge of the tub and place his foot onto a surface that has poor footing, will result in his fighting those staff. He is afraid of falling into the tub.

Having a resident balance on one leg as staff help him put on his pants, will result in some residents becoming aggressive. The staff know that they "have him", he doesn't.

In each of these examples, in order for the person being cared for to trust the staff doing the task he must know them and be familiar with their abilities. The mentally impaired do not know who is doing the care, their skill, nor can they remember what was done in the past. All the mentally impaired know is that someone is doing something to them. The more fearful the task, the more the potential loss of control, the greater the risk for an aggressive response in defense.

13. Progressive Agitation

Some residents are emotionally sensitive. It takes little to get them agitated. You walk into a resident's room to take him to the toilet, when a few moments before another resident was in his room swearing or going through his things. This build-up of emotion creates a low tolerance point that can easily result in an aggressive outburst if any further anxiety is created.

14. Old Behaviour
The resident may have been aggressive all of his life – it is normal for him to function that way. Swearing and a loud voice may have always been this person's way of dealing with stressful situations. Many tasks now are stressful, causing him to be loud and swearing during almost every contact.

15. Bombarding
The resident is being asked to do too much at one time. Getting up and eating breakfast may be stressful enough. If immediately after breakfast he is scheduled to have a bath, the added stress in such a short time span may be enough to set off an aggressive outburst.

Bombarding can also occur when too much verbal information is given at one time – "I want you to get up, put on your housecoat, eat your breakfast, then you can have a bath and go to your activity." We know all of that will be completed over a 2 hour period. To the resident it sounds as though it must all be done now. To avoid the pressure, the resident resists.

16. False Cuing
An important question that I pose to staff in long term care that just flabbergasts them is – "If I am mentally impaired, why is it okay to go to the bathroom in a chair by my bed, but not okay to go to the bathroom in a chair in the lounge?"

You are the one who knows that the chair by my bed is a commode chair with a hole in it. That is aptly called false cuing. Unless this person knows where he is, he will not know what it is you are asking him to do or the equipment you want him to use. I don't wash in my bed, I wash at a sink. I don't go to the toilet in my bed (bed pan or urinal), I go in the toilet. Some of the locations where we are performing care may not be the normal place for that task to be done. To the mentally impaired, the conflict results in a resistive reaction, which in turn can lead to an aggressive response.

Many things encountered by a resident can be confusing:

- – incontinent briefs – I need to go to the bathroom and I
  am going in my pants.
- – side rails up – I need to go to the bathroom and I can't
  get out of my bed.
- – a young girl is trying to take my pants off me
- – you are putting me to bed and other people are still up.
- – you are getting me up when it is still dark or you are
  putting me to bed when it is still light.

17. Personality Conflict

A mentally impaired resident may not get along with the staff member performing his care. This may have nothing to do with the staff member, but reflects the resident's perception. To this resident, that staff member reminds him of someone in his past that he disliked or didn't trust, or that staff member has an approach or a tone of voice, that for whatever reason the resident cannot tolerate. Dealing with that staff member only intensifies the resident's anxiety level to a panic state, causing an aggressive response.

18. Values

Having a female staff member care for a male resident or a male staff member care for a female resident may create an aggressive response in some. Again that is not always the case. It is not uncommon that certain female staff may be more effective in caring for certain male residents and certain male staff in caring for certain female residents.

Likewise an aggressive response can be initiated by the presence of visible minority staff (black, Chinese, etc.). If that older person had a long standing prejudice in the past, then it may be released now when such a staff member is in close proximity. That prejudice may be considered new to their family. Family may state that they never heard a racist slur by their parent until now. The reason for this apparent change in personality is straightforward. In the past mother had the ability to control and inhibit her comments. She consciously remained silent knowing that such beliefs about other races would not be well received or polite.

Now that she is mentally impaired, the ability to control or hide those beliefs is gone. Seeing "that person" now only intensifies her anxiety and she becomes aggressive.

19. Disease

It is very difficult to assess a mentally impaired resident's physical ability. A resident who is unable to communicate cannot state that his arthritis has limited his movement. It is difficult to know that his comfortable range of motion in his left shoulder has deteriorated to the point where his arm is parallel to the floor. Staff inadvertently raise his arm above his head when they help him put on his sweater. His response is to strike out whenever he is being dressed. Almost any disease process can effect a resident's ability to function including Alzheimer's, remember the resident can experience a volatile affect that makes him easily explosive.

AGGRESSION

Just dealing with this one behaviour is a complex issue. Determining what to do is even more complex. Without the process of Care Analysis, there can be little direction on how to effectively intervene with an individual demonstrating this behaviour.

When staff completed the Care Analysis process on Marg's behaviour, it was discovered that her aggressive outbursts may have been intensified by the following factors:

1. False Cuing – she was undressed and ready for bed when it was still daylight and the other residents on the unit were all dressed and up.
2. Approach – she was not supported by staff before, during or after any scheduled care task.
3. Timing – staff scheduled her care at a time when she had the greatest amount of energy and was able to provide the most resistance.

Through the analysis process, staff discovered that Marg's aggressive outbursts were just a symptom of a number of underlying problems that could be controlled. They found that if they dealt with these underlying problems, Marg's aggression would lessen.

The interventions in this case were as follows:

1. Prepare Marg for bed last (possibly as late as 2145 hours). Being tired, her ability to be aggressive would lessen, resulting in her going only "3" rounds instead of "13". Likewise the cuing would be supportive – by 2145 hours it would be dark outside and other residents would already be in bed or at least undressed and ready for bed.

2. Staff needed to ensure they had the time to be supportive – Staff were to ensure that when they performed care on Marg they would have the required time to provide the needed support before and after any procedures were completed.

Marg's behaviour of wandering the halls, pounding her fist and saying "they're stealing my clothes, they're stealing my clothes . . ." did not stop. Staff now encountered it from 9:45 PM until midnight instead of 5:00 PM until midnight (I would rather have two hours than seven – making the behaviour tolerable) and she was obviously less agitated by the change in approach and supportive tactics employed by the staff.

Prior to analyzing Marg's behaviour, staff just believed that this was just "Marg" – she is always aggressive and always would be – a "black/white" analysis.

The process of Care Analysis required the team to brainstorm and examine closely the complexity of this resident's behaviour. A necessary step when attempting to intervene on any resident behaviour in order to determine the most effective direction in resident care.

Care Analysis in summary involves the following:

1. On a flip chart provided, identification by the care team of the care issue encountered with this resident.
2. List all of the possible reasons why any mentally impaired resident may respond in that way.
3. Identify which of those reasons seems to best fit this resident.

Once a possible cause has been identified, it can be written as a Nursing Diagnosis for the resident care plan:

Aggressive when asked to perform care tasks –
Due to inappropriate approach and timing of task.

Once written in that manner, the interventions needed are obvious to all and from that point on are straightforward.

YOU MAY NOT STOP THE BEHAVIOUR

If the goal is to stop the resident's aggression, you may not be successful. I know only two ways to stop aggressive behaviour – restrain and/or sedate. Neither of these are very effective or acceptable interventions.

There is a further rationale to completing this type of analysis beyond simply providing direction in care and individualizing the care plan. It also effectively meets our mandate of providing a quality of life.

If through the process of care analysis, we identify that a resident becomes aggressive due to:

– a lack of privacy
– the inability to handle too many instructions or tasks at
one time (bombarding)
– an inappropriate approach

and all of the appropriate interventions are employed, the reality is that you may still never stop the resident's aggression.

By completing the analysis to determine these causative factors and setting up the necessary supports, you have achieved something very significant – whether this resident is aggressive or not, you have just established for him the most positive and supportive environment in which he can live, given his strengths and limitations at that time. The basis of Supportive Therapy. The essence for Quality of Life.

If that is not enough motivation for some, there is another reason to employ such an analytical technique. How much aggression will you encounter if you do not provide this resident with support in these areas? Lots! How much aggression will you encounter if you do provide this resident with support in these areas? Less! That is the main focus of any intervention with the mentally impaired elderly. It is not how do you stop the behaviour, but how do you lessen it so that it is tolerable. Remember, if a symptom of an Alzheimer's victim can be stopped with something other than medication, then it isn't Alzheimer's Disease that is causing it. The aggression is our problem, not hers. We need to decide how we will cope with it rather than expect to always eliminate it.

AGGRESSION IS NORMAL BEHAVIOUR

It is important to ensure with any care team that periodic verbal or physical aggressive outbursts by the mentally impaired elderly is normal behaviour. It may be the only way a mentally impaired resident can communicate to us what he wants.

You are mentally impaired
Sitting in your chair/
You do not want to move
You want to stay in that chair/
You are verbally unable to express what you want/

I enter
I take you by the elbow to stand you up/
You have no choice but to resist physically/
You refuse to stand up/
I persist/
The pressuring increases your anxiety level
You become aggressive/

If you are incapable of placing into thought what it is you want or incapable of constructing that thought into language, then you must communicate in the only way possible – resistance and aggression.

You will not stop the behaviour of many of the mentally impaired. Instead, we are challenged to continually determine if there are external factors that are within our control that intensify this person's aggressive outbursts. To establish the needed supports we must ensure that those factors are in check – the process of Care Analysis.

We will discuss the process of Care Analysis further in the next chapter involving Wandering.

APPROACH – Being in Control

This is probably the most appropriate time to discuss how to approach the mentally impaired. First it is necessary to ensure that we are discussing aggression as a symptom, not as a label. Aggression as a label implies that the person will be aggressive on every contact, all of the time, which is impossible. Aggression as a symptom indicates that aggression will be periodic, which is much more realistic.

It does not matter whether a mentally impaired resident has been aggressive in the past or not, staff must always expect that as a possible response. Just when you think you know what a mentally impaired resident will do, or how he will respond in a given situation, he will change it on you. To be effective with the mentally impaired, staff must always expect the unexpected. The resident's perceptions and abilities vary to such a significant degree from one situation to another, that he may respond positively to something at one time and become agitated to the same thing at another time. In order to maintain a safe setting when caring for this type of clientele, staff must always be prepared for a potential change in a resident's behaviour.

In fact when investigating situations where staff have been seriously injured by a mentally impaired resident, it is not uncommon for that injury to be the fault of the staff member herself. This is not to imply that staff are always the cause of a mentally impaired resident's aggression. We have already demonstrated that a variety of causes can create that one response. What is suggested is that a staff member's injury may have been avoided had that person taken the necessary steps to safeguard herself.

Imagine:

A potentially aggressive mentally impaired resident
Is sitting in a chair in the corner of a room/
A staff member steps into the corner
Beside the resident's chair/
She speaks down to the resident

Telling him she is going to help him stand up/
She takes him by the arm
The resident is surprised by the sudden contact/
He becomes startled/
His anxiety is elevated to a panic state
He stands and turns on the staff member/
Blocking the staff member in the corner
And starts hitting her/
What does she do?

We have all discovered the amazing strength that a mentally impaired resident can possess when he feels frightened or threatened. The staff member is now blocked into the corner and can only hope that someone will pull the resident off of her.

Approaching any mentally impaired resident must be a conscious, controlled effort by staff. Before any contact is made with any resident, staff must know that person's dominant side. The dominant side refers to whether the person is right handed or left handed. Once the dominant side has been discovered, then all contact is made from that side.

In the above scenario, the staff member needed to approach the resident in a very structured manner.

1. Approach at an angle on the dominant side (right side in this case). Being at an angle keeps herself in the person's field of vision (remember tunnel vision).
2. Crouch down to eye level so he can see her (if the stimulus is not intense enough, it will be missed or misinterpreted).
3. Place her right hand lightly on his right wrist and her right elbow lightly on his right knee, that touch will be sufficient stimuli to get his attention.
4. Talk to him for a short while to re–establish rapport.
5. Gradually raise him from the chair.

There is more to this approach than just being supportive. She has in effect restrained his movements. By placing her right hand on his right wrist and her right elbow on his right knee, the resident cannot make a move to strike her without her knowing it and controlling his actions.

The resident will not be conscious of being restrained. He does not possess the cognitive ability to immediately assess the situation and understand that her lightly touching him has that effect. Furthermore, he will not strike from the left side because of the effects of apraxia (the loss of purposeful muscle movements). His loss of coordination and muscle control makes movement from his non-dominant side awkward and weak. Besides the staff member is furthest away from that hand, and would have significant warning of the blow in order to move away and the blow itself would be weak having little effect. If he is going to strike, it will be from his strongest and most naturally dominant side, his right. Any movement made to attempt to strike would be immediately felt by the staff member allowing her to move away or deflect it. The staff member by approaching in this manner has made close, supportive contact, and also has been in control the entire time.

Staff must always be in control of a resident's dominant side, whether the person is sitting, lying in bed or walking down the hall. A staff member who approaches a mentally impaired resident walking down the hall from behind is only asking for trouble. To place a hand on a resident's shoulder from behind, when that person doesn't know you are there, creates a state called reality shock. The resident will be startled and might justifiably swing. To approach the same resident from the front is just as inappropriate. Standing in front of a mentally impaired resident who is walking down the hall results in blocking his path. He now is forced to stop or move around you. That forced change may result in his becoming agitated. Likewise to stand in front of him means that you must watch both his arms and legs, you are not in control of the situation and the potential of being injured if he strikes or kicks is high.

To approach a resident who is walking, staff must always approach that person at an angle on his dominant side. Staying at an angle keeps the staff member in the resident's field of vision, but does not block his progression forward. As you step close to him, you can place your left arm around his shoulder and your right hand lightly on his right wrist. The contact of your arm over his shoulder will get his attention and intensify rapport. Remember to read the behavioural cuing. If the resident pulls back, drops his shoulder when contact is made, or any other response to indicate he is not comfortable with the touch, withdraw your arm. By placing your right hand on his right wrist you are also in control of his dominant side. Should he become aggressive and attempt to swing, you can again either deflect the blow or step aside.

Working with the mentally impaired requires a variety of skills in order to be successful. Those who do not understand this clientele may believe that always being in control of a resident's dominant side is somewhat over-reactive. On the contrary, when a staff member does not employ this simple technique and is seriously injured, the results are more severe – the resident becomes labeled and is sedated.

It is our responsibility when caring for the mentally impaired to provide a controlled setting. We have demonstrated how that applies to admission and the environment, there is nothing different when discussing approach. Staff must always be in control of the situation for the resident's sake, as well as their own.

An easy way for staff to know quickly which side is that person's dominant is to establish on any unit that all residents are approached from the right side unless indicated differently.

RESIDENT ABUSE

Staff being in control is a major component for successful caring of the mentally impaired. That does not only apply to one's approach and the environment in which the care is completed, but to one's emotional state as well.

On one unit a young staff member was attempting to dress a mentally impaired resident. The resident was a "flailer", each time she was touched she began swinging her arms violently back and forth (another example of persistent stimuli). The staff member became frustrated with her inability to control the swinging arms and successfully dress the resident. The more she persisted to complete the task, the more intense was this resident's movements. The staff member finally lost control. She grabbed the resident by the wrists, squeezed them down to the armrests of the chair and yelled "I have had enough of you. Keep your arms still."

Had the pressure she applied to this resident been applied to your wrists, it would probably only have resulted in bruising. This lady was in her early eighties, with paper thin skin. The pressure the staff member applied was sufficient enough to create massive hematomas on both forearms that had to be lanced in order to relieve the pressure.

No matter the skills and compassion of any staff member, the mentally impaired have the ability to exhaust anyone's patience. The care is repetitive and at times can be exhausting. This will be experienced by the best of staff at one point or another. That is not what is being questioned here. We all have the ability to be pushed to our limit in any situation. What staff must be able to recognize is when that limit is reached. To have a staff member walk out of a resident's room and say to another staff member − "She is getting on my nerves, you take her for a while", is a strength. It shows that this person has the ability to walk away from a potentially stressful situation before it resulted in a regrettable outcome.

The young staff member who physically assaulted this resident did not recognize her limits. She lost control of the situation. All staff must know that there is virtually nothing they cannot walk away from when it concerns care − whether it is dressing a resident, washing that person, an activity and so on. It is more important to stay in control by stopping and do the task later or asking someone else to take over than the consequences of not taking either of those steps.

SUMMARY

There is nothing more disheartening than to have individuals over−simplify the behaviours of the mentally impaired. We have spent considerable time describing the complexities of this clientele, the gray areas that are not clearly visible, but must be enlightened in order to gain specific direction for intervention.

Your challenge is to demonstrate those complexities and insights to those who do not understand the mentally impaired. The process of Care Analysis is probably the most effective teaching tool that can be employed with any team. It teaches the team and its members the need to continually assess the mentally impaired in order to maintain the necessary objectivity to perform effective, personalized care.

Chapter Eleven

Wandering Behaviour

Care Analysis is effective in attempting to analyze any behaviour involving the mentally impaired. Wandering can now be discussed to the same intensity as we addressed aggressive behaviour.

First it is necessary to identify all of the possible reasons why a mentally impaired person may wander:

Mimicking
Looking for something familiar
Looking for (blank)
Fear/Anxiety/Stress
Bored
Poor Attention Span
Increased Energy
Medication/Washroom Location
Lifestyle
External Cuing
Physical Discomfort

1. Mimicking

Earlier we discussed how some mentally impaired residents can mimic almost any behaviour if the stimulus is intense enough. The same is true with wandering behaviour.

Defining the wandering path on a unit is a must. The wandering path is not only the physical layout of the unit, but the visible layout as well – the part of the hall or unit that attracts a mentally impaired resident to it.

If the wandering path takes or attracts a resident through a lounge, all you need to do is stand in the hall and watch the results. One wanderer will walk down the hall and into the lounge. Two mentally impaired residents will come out of the lounge and walk down the hall. On their return pass, they will both walk into the lounge. Three residents will then exit the lounge . . . Within a short time you could have up to six residents wandering all due to the activity of one.

Residents who are aware of the activity about them are the most susceptible. Such an individual can sit for extended periods of time if the environment is quiet and he is not distracted. If the wandering path is in view of this resident where he can see others walk past, then past again, he will be drawn to them. Once two residents are wandering the same path, others with a similar sensitivity to such activity are likely to follow.

The intervention required for this resident is to remove the wandering path from view of the lounge or remove the mimicker from view of the wanderer. In that way, this resident will not be attracted to follow the wanderer and will sit for extended periods.

2. Looking for Something Familiar

The need of some mentally impaired residents to find something familiar – spouse, house, clothing, etc., was presented earlier. To find something familiar is to make sense of the world you live in, decreasing the anxiety experienced. Wandering is in response to that need to be constantly looking.

3. Looking for (blank)

Some have called this activity mere curiosity on the part of the mentally impaired. There is more to it than that. This is the resident who has very poor recent memory retention. He does not know what he is looking for and neither do we. No matter what you give him, it does not satisfy him. His wandering may be his only way to understand the environment in which he lives.

> Being mentally impaired/
> I walk around the unit
> I come upon a door
> I can't remember what is behind that door
> So I open it/
> Once I see inside
> I know what it is/
> As I turn away from the door
> I immediately forget about it/
>
> I wander around the unit again

I come upon the same door
I don't remember what is behind it
So I look again/
Once I look
I remember/

I wander around the unit
I come upon the same door . . ./

This resident is continually investigating the environment. The degree of recent memory loss prevents him from remembering what he has just seen. As soon as he looks behind a door or in a drawer, he understands what he is looking at and feels secure with that knowledge. As soon as he turns around, he forgets what he has seen. To attempt to remember and make sense of where he is, he must keep wandering and looking. Wandering is a way of maintaining some control and sense of order over the environment.

Each of these cases – looking for something familiar and looking for (blank), can be called random wandering. Whenever a mentally impaired resident gets it in his mind that he must find something, he will wander. The best thing to do is to let that resident wander. To stop him is to increase his anxiety and increase the possibility of an aggressive response. When he cannot wander he feels more confused, which will elevate his anxiety. To wander gives him the feeling that he knows what is going on around him. Allowing a mentally impaired resident to wander freely requires a safe wandering environment (discussed at length later in this chapter).

There is one intervention that is sometimes effective to break this person's wandering pattern, it is called diversionary activity. It may be necessary to periodically intervene on this person's wandering when the activity on the unit is too much, he is disturbing others, or the resident himself is becoming exhausted and must be encouraged to sit in order to rest. Employing a diversionary activity is an attempt to take the resident's mind off whatever he is looking for. That activity may keep him occupied for 20 minutes one day and the very next day you are lucky the same activity will occupy him for 20 seconds. His concentration depends on the degree of his anxiety at the time.

206

4. Fear/Stress/Anxiety

I am a mentally impaired resident
Living in a long term care facility/
You approach me and take me to the lounge/
You sit me in a chair
Next to me is a female resident who is mentally impaired/

When you leave/
The resident next to me
Places her hands all over me/
I do not know who she is or that she is impaired
All I know is that I experience considerable anxiety from
      her actions/
I wander out of the lounge in response/

This may only happen on a few occasions,
Over time
As soon as I am placed in the lounge/
Whether that resident is there or not/
I wander out/
Sit me in any other room and I will remain for an extended
      period of time/

Some residents may refuse to sit in a certain lounge due to negative experiences encountered with that room. That lounge now has associated with it considerable fear causing a need to wander when placed there. The resident will remember only what he is able to remember. Faces mean nothing, therefore he will now associate his fear with the room, a conditioned response.

The resident who can wash himself at the side of the bed, but cannot handle tub time may be seen wandering between 0830 and 1130 hours every morning. Depending on his cognitive ability and his awareness of things around him, seeing staff use the tub, talking about baths and getting bath equipment may elicit a response from him "My turn is next". Once the bath things are put away, he settles and his wandering stops, again a conditioned response.

Likewise the resident who has his arm pulled by a specific staff member when being taken to the bathroom is at greatest risk of wandering when that staff member is on duty.

In each of these cases, it is a specific stressor that is causing this person's wandering behaviour. Eliminate the stressor and you will find that the wandering will be curtailed.

This shows the difference between working with the cognitively well versus the mentally impaired. If a cognitively well resident experiences difficulty with his situation or environment, that person can be asked what is bothering him. The mentally impaired often do not provide such direct feedback. To ask a level two mentally impaired resident what is bothering him will often provide little useful information. This person is usually unable to accurately assess his situation and has difficulty communicating clearly what is disturbing him.

We have just identified an important aspect of understanding the mentally impaired and defining the concepts employed in caring for this clientele. First, if you leave a mentally impaired resident to solve his own problems, the solution will always be inappropriate. Secondly, even though the mentally impaired cannot communicate directly, they always communicate indirectly through their behaviour. It is his behaviour that will demonstrate his distress.

Wandering caused by a specific stressor can be aptly called patterned. Patterned wandering occurs virtually the same time every day. It is important to identify patterned wandering in order to determine the necessary intervention.

If staff suspect that a resident begins his wandering at a specific time each day, they must then initiate steps to define the pattern. The rationale for defining the pattern is to uncover the stressor that is elevating the resident's anxiety level and take the necessary steps to eliminate it. To accomplish this, the care team must monitor the resident's wandering during specified shifts over a two week period. That requires all team members (housekeeping, activity staff, nursing, etc.) to observe and record the wandering activity of that resident for that shift. When the resident is seen wandering, then the staff member who discovered him must chart the time and "back track", describing what was occurring in the last location where he was sitting (an activity, aggressive outbursts, bright room, etc.).

By reviewing what is charted, staff may uncover a trend that will demonstrate what is causing this resident difficulty, for example:

On four occasions when the resident was observed, he was found wandering each time around 1400 hours. When staff "back tracked" or described where he was sitting last, it was always the lounge and on each occasion an activity scheduled for 1330 hours was just wrapping up.

On further investigation it was discovered that this resident was not directly involved in that activity. This suggests that he may be unable to handle the stimuli created by that event. The noise and movement by those involved in the activity increases his anxiety level causing his need to wander. In order to intervene on this resident's behalf, it is then necessary for staff to remove him from the lounge before the activity begins or to re-locate the activity to another room.

Always finding the stressor or cause for the person's wandering may not be so easy. The descriptions by staff of where the resident was last sitting may indicate no obvious pattern in activity or stimuli to reveal the possible stressor. What this exercise can identify that is very helpful is the time pattern. If the resident was found to wander everyday around 1400 hours, then a diversional activity of some type would be beneficial at that time. It makes little sense to have this resident scheduled for an activity in the morning when he would sit content in the lounge, and nothing at 1400 hours when he has difficulty with something on the unit. Scheduling an activity at 1400 hours for this resident removes him from the stressor experienced on the unit even though it has not been uncovered.

5. Bored, Poor Attention Span, Increased Energy Level

These are all related. A resident with poor recent memory may also have a poor attention span and as a result an increased energy level. This individual easily loses track of what is happening, finding most activities or events confusing. This results in his becoming bored, increasing his restlessness, encouraging him to wander.

To understand a contributing factor in causing this wandering activity, we need only examine the activity department and its programming. Most long term care facilities have a limited number of activity staff, a common ratio is 1 to 50, one activity staff member to every 50 residents. Such a high ratio does not allow activity staff much of an opportunity for one-to-one programming. As a result, an exercise program may last 20 to 30 minutes and have 10 or more residents involved.

Imagine:

> You are running an exercise program
> There are ten residents participating/
> Six are cognitively well, physically disabled
> Three are high functioning mentally impaired
> Able to concentrate/
> One resident who is also mentally impaired
> Who has a very limited attention span/
>
> You begin the exercises/
> Three minutes into the program
> One of the mentally impaired residents wanders out/
> You have two options/
> Continually stall the group
> Dragging back the resident with a limited attention span/
> Or let her go
> To spend your time with the other residents/
>
> What would you do?

The most common response is to let her go. That means the person who needs the activity the most may be the one who gets it the least.

The mentally impaired who suffer from a poor attention span can only concentrate on something for 4 minutes or less, after which he becomes bored and restless. His inability to concentrate any longer on what is happening results in his standing and walking away. If the wandering path in which he walks is complicated, with many blind bluffs and turns, he can easily become confused. Not knowing where he is going, he then sits in the first empty chair he can find. Again he only sits in that chair for about 4 minutes, not remembering why he is there, he becomes bored and restless, stands and begins to wander again. Finding the first empty chair he comes to, he sits . . . He continues that activity throughout the day. This type of wandering can be aptly called Stop/Go Wandering.

Again if you leave a mentally impaired resident to solve his own problem, the solution will always be inappropriate. This resident is responding to his restlessness by moving from one chair to another. His activity does not exhaust his increasing energy level and as a result does nothing to alleviate his problem. The only practical intervention for this resident is to provide bursts of activity every hour to an hour and a half, in order to decrease his restlessness and eliminate the need for the stop/go wandering.

A common response by some managers and staff to such a suggestion is that it cannot be done. Time and staffing restraints make it impossible to implement such an intervention. Their assessment of the actual situation is totally inaccurate. On most units such tactics are employed, but unfortunately not consistent. It often depends who is on duty at the time, whether it is done or not.

If the right housekeeper is on duty, one who understands the mentally impaired, she is often doing what is required. You will find that the housekeeper usually cleans the resident's lounge the first thing in the morning when few residents are there. The residents who are in the lounge are usually the one's who become restless easily, and wakes up by 0430 hours. The staff who discover them at that time, get them up and dressed rather than attempting to force them to stay in bed and sleep. That means those residents could have been sitting in the lounge for an extended period of time before the housekeeper walks in to clean. If that housekeeper is one who can relate well to the mentally impaired, she will always go beyond her basic duties. If she notices that certain residents are becoming restless while she is in the lounge, she will turn on the radio and get them singing and dancing at the same time she is cleaning. That housekeeper has just provided the needed burst of activity to decrease the restlessness of those residents and prevented their need to wander.

The same is true when it comes to certain nursing staff. If the right staff member is on duty, she is usually providing bursts of activity to the residents who need it. She will often encourage specific residents to follow her at certain times of the day, asking them to carry laundry or push a cart under supervision. That staff member knows that <u>making</u> those residents sit in the lounge for extended periods will only cause them to become restless and possibly even agitated, effecting the ability to perform care as the day progresses. This is sound problem solving on the part of certain staff.

What is interesting is to listen to the criticism this staff member will receive by those staff who do not understand the rationale for what she is doing – "Stop babying her", "Quit spoiling her." A totally inappropriate interpretation of what is being done. This is <u>effective programming</u>. This staff member is intervening on a resident's behaviour when it is needed, rather than waiting until the person demonstrates a serious behavioural problem.

Residents cannot afford hit/miss programming, where it depends who is on as to what is being done. It is important that the care team identify the residents that fit this criteria – low attention span, easily bored, high energy. Once identified, those residents are then scheduled to have bursts of activity throughout their day. That means that if the housekeeper is in the lounge at 0700 hours and those specific residents are there, then she is responsible to get them moving at that time for about 5 minutes. Likewise, nursing staff need to spread out their care routine, so that breakfast, bathing and other activities are not done between 0800 and 0900 hours and the resident is left alone until lunch. Doing one care task each hour through the morning accomplishes the desired results. Furthermore, recreation staff must be asked to sprinkle throughout the day five minutes of exercises for these residents when no other activity is scheduled. These exercise sessions can be coordinated well with activity staff, volunteers, family members and staff of other departments. This simple scheduling method ensures that during every hour to an hour and a half these resident have something that exhausts their energy level, decreasing their restlessness and possibly eliminating much of the stop/go wandering.

6. The Disease Process

This may again be the persistent stimuli effect, where this resident cannot stop walking. The only thing that stops this resident from wandering is pure exhaustion, which will result in frequent falls. The best intervention in this case is to have staff check this resident every two hours to see if she is getting tired and having difficulty keeping up the pace. If it is obvious she is tired, then staff will have no choice but to restrain her in a chair for a period so she can rest. Even in the chair her legs will be continually moving.

Watch out for structure! The standard practice may be to keep her in a chair for up to an hour, then to let her out of the chair so she can resume her walking. If she begins fighting the restraint after 45 minutes, she is telling you that her energy is back and it is time to let her go, checking her again in another hour. Unfortunately, when some staff see her fighting the restraint, they will respond "You can't get up, you're supposed to stay in that chair for another 15 minutes." When they finally let her up, they now have an aggressive wanderer on their hands.

7. Medications & Location of The Washroom

Two drugs that can cause wandering are diuretics and laxatives. We have already identified the sensitivity of the mentally impaired elderly to medication. It does not matter which biological process the medication works on, the effects are the same. A mentally impaired resident on a laxative or diuretic will always have the feeling that "he has to go". If he is aware of the need and fear of being incontinent, he will continually wander in order to find the washroom. The problem is that when he finds it, he does not need it at that time, so he keeps wandering until he does.

Unfortunately, the location of the washroom itself can cause wandering. If there are many doors to choose from and none are clearly marked, then the resident must wander until he finds the room that looks like a washroom.

8. Lifestyle

It has been said "If you have marital problems, you are supposed to sit down and talk them out." It seems in my Dad's and Grandfather's day, they didn't sit down and talk it out, they stood up and walked it out, always having an excuse to walk around the block or around the "back forty" when things got too tense.

An important question to ask the family of a mentally impaired resident is "How has your dad dealt with stress all of his life?" Their answer will provide considerable insight into dad's behaviour now. If family indicate that their father has always dealt with stress in the past by walking it off, then that is probably what he is doing now by his constant wandering. It is important then to let him wander.

Likewise, past history may indicate another motivator for a resident's wandering. One unit had a male resident who demonstrated chronic and sometimes agitated wandering. All efforts by staff to distract him from his incessant, non–directed wandering failed until family revealed an interesting point about their dad's past. The only history staff had on this resident was that he had been a labourer for the past 38 years. Family revealed months after dad's admission that their father really had been a sweeper for the past 20 years. Wandering was his life.

Immediately upon receiving that information, the staff on that unit gave this resident a broom and encouraged him to sweep the hallway. From that point on, his wandering became directed and his agitation was completely eliminated. Each day he would find some debris on the floor and chase it around the unit with his broom. More importantly, he was now more cooperative to stop for his lunch and by late afternoon he could be persuaded to put his broom away and sit in the lounge for a period of time. If during the evening he saw some dirt in the hallway, he would get his broom, chase it around the unit for awhile and then return his broom back to its closet. Staff successfully change what was before a disruptive behaviour to something that was now tolerable.

A further footnote about this gentleman. He often displayed another interesting behaviour – now when you stop him while he is sweeping to have a brief conversation, he will stand with his right elbow leaning on his broom and his left hand stroking his chin ("old behaviour", something he had probably done for the 20 years that he was a sweeper).

9. External Cuing

There is one season that can create a significant amount of wandering activity on any unit, it is spring. We all know what it is like to be cooped up indoors all winter and then experience a beautiful April day. Our own desire to be out in the sun may even cause us to wander outdoors every opportunity we have, not unlike the power such a day has on certain mentally impaired residents within the facility.

The time of the day can also entice some mentally impaired residents to wander. The most common occurrence on some units may be at the change of shift. It depends how staff leave the unit. If the day staff all congregate at the nursing station and all leave the unit like "a heard of charging elephants", then they will probably be taking a number of mentally impaired residents with them. The stimulus such a commotion creates may be intense enough to now entice some residents to want to "go home". On the other hand, if staff leave the unit one at a time, where it is hardly noticed that there is a transition to the next shift, then wandering at that time will probably be less.

10. Physical Discomfort

How many of our residents have arthritis? A person with arthritis can only sit for a certain period of time until he finds it necessary to move or else stiffen up. Physical pain, constipation, wanting something to eat may all cause a person to wander in order to satisfy any of those needs.

DEALING WITH WANDERING BEHAVIOUR

Some will say "Why not just let all of the residents who want to wander, wander?" In some situations that is the most appropriate intervention. The decision to intervene on wandering behaviour depends on what is causing it. Like aggression and almost all other behaviours of the mentally impaired, wandering may be a symptom of an underlying problem as demonstrated above. The intervention needed depends on the problem causing it.

For some residents, there is no intervention available that will stop or decrease their wandering, and for others there is. Excessive wandering by a number of residents on any unit can create significant problems:

1. Mimic wandering – residents who are capable of concentrating on a specific task can be distracted by the constant stimuli of seeing others wander and as a result are unable to complete the task.
2. Indiscriminate wandering – you cannot control a large number of residents who wander all at one time. There will be constant wandering into other resident's rooms and

rummaging through other resident's things which will
increase the incidents of aggressive outbursts on the unit
3. Lineal wandering – walking up and down a hall with no
change in direction is more like pacing than wandering
and can cause an increase in anxiety, increasing agitation.
4. Increased risk of elopement behaviour – the more residents
that are wandering, the more who are attempting to leave
the building.
5. Forced wandering – the more residents wandering, the
greater risk that some residents will be virtually dragged
out of their chairs by wandering residents wanting them to
follow, increasing the incidents of aggressive outbursts
and placing a not too stable resident at risk of falling.

The list goes on. Wandering on the unit must be safe and
controlled so that it is not in excess, does not disrupt other
residents and will not result in the person being injured or injuring
others. To accomplish this, there are a number of options that can
be employed when dealing with wandering behaviour.

1. The Physical Wandering Path

The most appropriate wandering path is one that provides
directional change. Any unit that is shaped in a "U" or in a circle
would accomplish that effect. Directional change eliminates from
the wanderer an awareness that he is covering the same territory
over and over again. Lineal wandering or wandering up and down
a straight corridor, can be akin more to pacing or a "caged in"
feeling, which can increase agitation.

If the unit can only provide a lineal wandering path, then
the responsibility is on staff to define the resident's endurance
level (how long before the wanderer becomes agitated). Some
mentally impaired residents can wander back and forth on such a
unit every day, all day long and not experience any difficulty.
Others can tolerate pacing the hall for only a short time before
they feel trapped, increasing their anxiety to a panic level, causing
an agitated response.

When it is discovered that a resident can only tolerate
wandering on a lineal unit for no longer than an hour before he
becomes agitated, then staff must intervene. They need to
schedule some type of activity and spread out their care routine to

216

cover every hour to allow a break in that resident's wandering. As discussed earlier, such an intervention strategy would involve all departments and a re-scheduling of the care routine to ensure that this resident is taken away from the hall every hour to do something else.

2. Defining The Wandering Path

It is important to clearly define the wandering path on any unit. This can be accomplished by a number of means. A tiled hallway floor can have the centre tiles removed and replaced with a brightly coloured tile. In essence you are creating a path in the floor that may literally outline for the resident what direction to take (like following the yellow brick road). Such a path prevents some residents from taking the wrong direction into alcoves or other rooms.

That same concept can be applied to hand rails as well. Painting hand rails a bright colour along the path you want the residents to follow makes that direction stand out, steering the resident around the unit.

It is important on any unit to conceal at least one of the lounges from the wanderer to protect the resident who will mimic such activity. To accomplish this, just place a louvred paneled wall in front of the entrance to a lounge. The location of that panel must not block the hallway or impede exiting from the lounge. By obscuring the entrance to the lounge, you have created a significant deterrent that will prevent the wanderer from walking in and out of the lounge, drawing out the mimicker. Placing the louvers at an angle allows staff to see into the lounge, but looks like a solid wall when the wanderer walks straight towards it.

3. Creating a Safe Wandering Environment

Elopement behaviour is the attempt by a mentally impaired resident to leave the building. There are two types of elopement behaviour. One is the direct eloper, this is the resident who makes a "bee line" for the nearest exit and once outside is difficult to return to the building. The other is indirect eloper, the resident who is found wandering aimlessly out in the yard and is easy to return to the unit.

A common cause creating the indirect eloper is that the resident is attracted out of the building by something he has seen. If an exit door is in direct view from the wandering path, allowing the wanderer to see outside through the window in that door, he may be drawn out by: a nice sunny day, a shopping mall down the street, a garden that needs to be tended, people walking along the sidewalk, etc. He is not intending to leave but just drawn outside. Once outside, the door locks when it closes behind him, he cannot return inside, so he wanders aimlessly until someone takes him back in.

The same occurs if a wandering resident can see a stairwell as he walks past a door. Once he sees the stairs, he will go down for a simple reason – to see where they go (the mentally impaired are always looking for something familiar and investigating the environment to decrease their anxiety). By the way you will rarely find a mentally impaired resident going up the stairs, you will more often find him going down. That is due to progressive apraxia. To go up the stairs requires considerable muscle coordination and strength. To go down the stairs, one just flows with gravity.

There are two successful interventions that can be employed in each of these cases. One way is to use smoked glass coverings or sheers over the door windows. Anyone entering the unit through those doors is able to see through the darkened glass or sheers to ensure that no one is standing behind the door before they open it. The darkened glass will appear solid black to the mentally impaired, keeping the exterior or stairwells from view, decreasing the tendency to be drawn through the door.

One of the best ways to ensure safe wandering is to secure exterior and stairwell doors. Buzzers are of little value. It is the time you don't check the door that the resident you were afraid was going to leave has left. A magnetic security device solves many problems. The magnetic security device works on the same principle as the magnetic fire door closures. Fire doors in hallways of most facilities are propped open against electronic magnets on the walls. The magnet, when it is activated, holds the fire doors open, allowing easy access and ventilation. The source of power to those magnets is connected to the fire alarm system. When the fire alarm sounds or the power goes off, the magnets automatically shut off, releasing the fire doors and they close tight.

The magnetic security device works under the same principle, but in reverse. An electronic magnet attached to the door frame of an exit door holds the door closed. When someone wants to leave or enter the unit, that person needs to push in and hold a button on the wall. Once the button is pressed, it deactivates the magnet and releases the door, allowing the person to open the door. Once the button is released, the magnet is reactivated automatically, securing the door as soon as it closes.

The power to this magnet is also connected to the fire alarm system. When the fire alarm sounds or the power goes off, the magnet is deactivated and the door can be opened freely. With this device, the door is not locked, but only secured, making it nearly impossible for the mentally impaired to open it and leave the unit.

Another security device that is even more complex is the numbered magnetic security system. It works on the same principle as what was just described. The difference is that instead of having one button, there is a box with six buttons each numbered from one to six. A person coming onto the unit needs to only turn the handle on the door, the magnet is automatically deactivated. To leave the unit, you must push specific numbers in sequence on the box. Once the appropriate sequence is pressed, the magnet is deactivated, and the door will open freely. Again, if the fire alarm sounds or the power goes off, the magnet automatically shuts off and the door can be opened freely.

To allow visitors, family members, cognitively well residents and other staff to freely come and go from the unit, it is important to place a sign just below the deactivating button with instructions on how to open the door. A mentally impaired resident will be unable to read the instructions, understand what they mean, push the button and have the manual dexterity to open the door at the same time. If that resident is capable of following those instructions and open the door, then I question his degree of impairment.

One last point on using this device. If the button that deactivates the lock is a black button, surrounded by a silver wall cover, located on a brown wall, then you will have some problems. Some of your mentally impaired residents will be attracted to that wall plate, pushing it over and over again (if the stimulus is too intense, some mentally impaired cannot help but respond). A simple solution is to wallpaper the wall, over the silver cover, with a pattern of black eyed Suzies. To the mentally impaired the button is lost in a sea of black buttons (if the stimulus is not intense enough it will be missed or misinterpreted) and they are no longer attracted to it.

One last point on creating a safe wandering path. The wanderer must have available to him visible resting areas scattered throughout. These could be small alcoves where a couple of comfortable chairs and a small end table are located. In this way the wanderer is provided an opportunity to rest during his journey.

4. Securing an Elevator

It is always interesting to see the colour elevators are painted on units that house the mentally impaired. Often the walls are beige and the elevator is bright blue. That is exactly what we discussed to make resident rooms stand out – paint the door frames a bright colour in contrast to the wall. To hide the elevator, it need only be painted the same colour as the wall. That will make it virtually invisible, preventing the mentally impaired from being attracted to it.

The elevator will still be a problem. On the wall next to the elevator is a steel plate with two buttons. The mentally impaired will be attracted to the plate and buttons, pushing one often by accident. The elevator is summoned, the door opens, the resident is attracted inside the elevator, the door closes, the elevator proceeds to the next floor, the door opens again and the resident walks out wandering about on another floor.

A simple intervention is to have maintenance staff place a metal plate secured to the wall, covering the two buttons. Two holes are pre-drilled in the plate, one over each of the buttons. The holes must be smaller than an adult's little finger. Next to the plate, anchored to the wall is a small chain attached to the end of it. The stick is the exact diameter of the holes in the plate. To summon the elevator, one only needs to slip the stick through one of the holes and depress the button. The mentally impaired will be unable to use such a complex device. They can no longer summon the elevator on their own.

Two interventions have been presented, one that prevents the mentally impaired from being drawn to the elevator by its colour, and the other by accidentally summoning the elevator by pushing the buttons. A third potential problem still remains where the elevator opens on its own as a mentally impaired resident walks by. If someone summoned the elevator and walked away or if there are two elevators and both come to the unit when the button is pushed, the resident sees the doors open and inadvertently walks in. What is needed to prevent this is a black mat placed on the floor in front of the elevator.

Some have tried these mats in front of exit doors, but found that they are usually not successful. The rationale for using the black mat is based on the perceptual difficulties experienced by the mentally impaired. Many mentally impaired residents have difficulty interpreting colour changes experienced on the floor. One facility demonstrated this well. The hall consisted of white floor tiles with a black border lining the wall. The black border ran across the entrance to the dining room. Staff found that they had considerable difficulty getting certain mentally impaired residents to cross the threshold into the dining room. When these residents reached the door and saw the black strip, they would stop, requiring staff to coax them to continue. When the resident proceeded through the door, he would inadvertently raise his foot to step over the black line. Those black lines represented a hole or a step (if the stimulus is not intense enough, it will be missed or misinterpreted) and the resident was unsure of how to cross over.

The black mat creates the same effect. If placed in front of an exit door, it may stall the mentally impaired from proceeding, but it will not stop them. They will reach the mat, place one foot on it to test it, then another foot and another until they reach the door. When placed in front of an elevator the black mat is most effective. The resident is walking past the elevator just as the doors are opening. The person turns to walk in, sees the mat and stops. Not sure of what it is, he will take one step on the mat to test it, then another and another. By the time he reaches the elevator door, it will have closed and he will walk away.

DEALING WITH DIRECT ELOPEMENT BEHAVIOUR

There are few mentally impaired residents who are true direct elopers. The direct eloper is one who heads for any exit door he can find and makes a "bee line" down the street. It is interesting to watch some staff attempt to deal with this individual. Once the resident has left the building, two staff will run after him. They come up from behind the resident, grab him by the arm and attempt to turn him around to lead him back to the facility. His response is to become aggressive for a number of reasons. Even though he is mentally impaired, he still knows that he is being turned around. Seeing two staff (people he does not know) virtually attack him will only result in his defending himself.

When staff discover that a resident has walked away from the building, their strategy must be well planned. If two staff may be needed, one should approach the resident from one side of the street and another from the opposite side. When the one on the same side of the street reaches the resident, she must circle around to the resident's dominant side and approach at an angle to be in his field of vision and not block his path. That staff member needs to smile at the resident and carry on a conversation that will relax him and enhance rapport. The other staff member should only approach the resident when called upon. The resident must then be guided around the block and back to the facility. The mentally impaired will not be aware of returning to the facility when taken around the block. This approach strongly increases the likelihood of returning to the facility with the least amount of aggression.

It is important that the care team use the eloper's exiting as an excuse to assess the environment. If it was that easy for a resident to leave the building, then steps must be taken to adapt the environment to prevent it from occurring again (as discussed earlier).

SUMMARY

Those who believe little can be done to assist the mentally impaired lack a great deal of imagination. To be effective with this clientele is to be creative, a risk taker – coming up with an idea or an approach, then implementing it to see if it is successful and continually evaluating it to determine its appropriateness. The more that staff can be encouraged to analyze and problem solve, the more appropriate and effective their care.

Determining what needs to be done for each specific resident is not a haphazard process. It requires considerable skill and energy. The only interventions that are successful are those that have undergone an effective assessment of the client's strengths and limitations – the basis of Supportive Therapy.

Chapter Twelve

Assessment

Appropriate and effective assessment is essential to determine the approach and interventions needed to effectively care for the mentally impaired elderly. The assessment process involves a number of different areas:

1. Medical
2. Environmental
3. Functional (ADL, social, activity, etc.)
4. Psychological Profile
5. Mental Status
6. History
7. Medication

THE ASSESSMENT PROCESS

Many long term care facilities have encountered problems in finding assessment mechanisms that are useful to the direct caregiver. The factors that seem to make the assessment process less than adequate include the following:

1. Those involved in the care are not directly involved in the assessment process.
2. The assessment mechanisms used are often of a diagnostic nature rather than a functional one.
3. The forms and process used are often taken directly from other sources (books, other facilities, etc.) without being adapted to the facility's resources and needs.

If those staff who are to use the information cannot understand what the assessment is supposed to identify or how the information is related to their care, then the findings will be filed in the chart and rarely referred to by the direct line staff. An effective assessment mechanism is one that is practical to the people doing the care and requires their involvement for its completion.

The purpose of assessment is to define the strengths and weaknesses of a mentally impaired resident and provide direction for the appropriate supports needed. No one assessment form can accomplish all of that and no form used by one facility can be totally effective for another. The needs of each facility vary depending on the facility's resources, staff training, the programs available, the physical environment of the building, the number and functioning level of the resident population, etc. There is little value in completing 30 questions on an assessment form developed by another facility, when the answers of only 16 questions are used in this facility. The only effective assessment mechanism is the one that the facility develops based on what it has to work with and what information it needs.

It is not necessary for a facility to work from scratch in developing such a form, but only to examine the various forms available, and then pulling from them what is useful in your facility. There have been a number of assessment procedures identified throughout this text, and in the next few pages even more will be highlighted. Use these along with the other assessment forms you have in your facility to develop an assessment process that provides the information you need relative to your situation.

Earlier chapters discussed the medical, environmental and mental status assessments. We will now review the medication, functional, history and the psychological profile assessments.

MEDICATION ASSESSMENT

The difficulties we experience with the mentally impaired in relation to medication usage stems from a number of sources:

1. At times the treating physician is not the resident's original doctor.
2. The original symptom that initiated ordering a specific drug may no longer be present.
3. Those who influence the ordering of medication may not be experienced with specific residents and their behaviours.

4. The functional ability and behaviour of many mentally impaired residents can change given certain circumstances and time.
5. Specific drugs may have a gradual build-up to toxic levels over time.
6. A long standing drug may now create problems when combined with another agent.
7. The tolerance level of the mentally impaired to medication may be substantially less than the general population of older people.

In working with the mentally impaired elderly, the best approach in regards to medication is "when in doubt, do without". To ensure that the medications used are the most appropriate, three specific assessment mechanisms are needed:

a) Ongoing Assessment
b) Three Month Review
c) Trial Period Without

A) Ongoing Assessment

The sensitivity of the mentally impaired to medication is an ongoing concern. It is essential for staff at all levels to report changes noted in a resident's behaviour or ability – drowsiness, altered gait, loss in muscle coordination, etc.

Some medications can cause a gradual build-up, where toxic effects are not demonstrated until the drug has been administered for a considerable period. It is the direct line staff who can best monitor a resident's functioning ability from one day to the next. Line staff must understand their role in monitoring drug use with this clientele. Even though their knowledge of specific drugs may be limited, their assessment is crucial. All staff must be encouraged to vocalize suspected changes in a resident's functioning and allowed to question whether a drug is helping or hindering a resident's abilities.

The care conference is the ideal vehicle for such questions and concerns. Encouraging staff's input can be accomplished by tapping their intuitive assessment ability of whether the medication is useful or not.

B) Three Month Drug Review

As mentioned above, the best philosophy concerning drug usage is "when in doubt, do without". Given the sensitivity of this clientele to medication, regular monitoring by the physician and care team is essential. Considering we know very little about the effects of one drug on any one resident, a combination of 6, 8 or 10 in a 24 hour period becomes a major concern.

A commonly used drug assessment process is the Three Month Drug Review. In order to ensure that this review has some clout and drugs are not simply rewritten every three months without being scrutinized, a policy must be established that dictates an automatic stop order on all drugs every three months.

Any drug can be re-ordered but it must be treated as a new order. This requires the physician to not only write the order on the Doctor's Order Sheet, but also write the reason the drug is to be continued in the Doctor's Progress Notes. This can be simplified. Drugs related specifically to a resident's diagnosis are easily dealt with. If the resident is on Aldomet for hypertension and Diabeta for diabetes, then he simply writes in the doctor's progress notes:

Aldomet (see medical)
Diabeta (see medical)

The drugs being challenged by this process are the non-life threatening medications such as the hypnotics and sedatives. These are drugs that have been ordered primarily to deal with behavioural issues.

When reviewing any medication, one simple question needs to be asked of the physician before he re-writes the order:

"Doctor, what would happen if we took that drug and decreased the dosage or stopped the drug all together?"

If he answers "You can't do that or this will happen . . .", he has just given the rationale for why that drug must be continued. If he answers "I don't know!", then he has just initiated the next assessment tool required – the Trial Period Without.

227

C) The Trial Period Without

If, a mentally impaired resident demonstrates considerable aggressive behaviour and frequently attempts to leave the building on admission does it mean that after 6 months of living on the unit he will still be aggressive and attempt to leave the building?

(Note: It is assumed in discussing this case that all necessary measures have been taken to determine that the aggressive and elopement behaviour demonstrated cannot be controlled by any other intervention other than medication.)

There are three possible answers. One, is he is worse. His aggressive outbursts and attempts to leave have increased since admission. In that case no medication has been found to be effective, and you have been testing different types of drugs, dosages, etc. with no success. There is no use considering that person for the Trial Period Without.

Another possible scenario is that this resident's aggression seems to have leveled, where the medication being dispensed is just holding him under control. He is still having periodic outbursts, but it is considered by all to be too early to take this resident off his medication.

The possibility is just as high that this resident would no longer be aggressive or attempt to leave the building, even if he were off the medication. The aggressive and elopement behaviour may no longer be present for two reasons. The first is that the disease may have progressed to the point that he no longer has the ability to be aggressive. The second is that he may have gained sufficient familiarity with the staff, routines and unit over the past six months to decrease his anxiety level and eliminate the aggressive response. In either case, why is he still on the original medication ordered to control that behaviour?

A very effective assessment mechanism to determine if specific non–life threatening medications – sedatives, hypnotics, anti–anxiety agents, etc. are still needed is the Trial Period Without. If over the last 2 months there has not been a recurrence of the original symptoms that initiated the medication, or the physician does not know the effect if a dosage is lowered or the drug is discontinued, then the resident is tried without that drug or with a lower dose for a period of four to eight weeks (the appropriate length will depend on the half life of the specific medication). It is advisable that a back–up prn sedative be ordered during this time if necessary. If there is no behavioural change during the trial period, then the medication is discontinued or the dosage is decreased further. Once there is some indication of a behavioural change (increased restlessness, greater difficulty to complete care tasks, etc.), then the drug can be elevated slightly, indicating that the most therapeutic dose for this resident has been reached.

It is important when implementing such a program that one medication be attempted at a time. If two or more drugs are experimented with and specific behaviours recur, it will be impossible to determine which drug is needed and which is not.

It is crucial that all staff be involved in the resident's behavioural and functional assessment during the trial perio̊. Having a resident in a full blown agitated state 8 days after the drug has been decreased or removed, requires considerable energies and resources to calm him and negatively impacts the rest of the unit. Direct line staff (aides, housekeepers, activity staff, etc.) must report any changes observed – increased restlessness, difficult to toilet, harder to perform personal care, unable to sit for any length of time, etc., when they occur.

The information provided by direct line staff is important for two reasons. First, identifying any subtle changes in behaviour may provide the necessary warning of a potential increase in agitation that may require the medication to be re–instated. Secondly, it helps to determine if there is any improvement in the resident's functioning or behaviour now that the medication has been decreased or stopped.

Summary of Trial Period Without

1. The behaviour that initiated ordering the medication has not been seen within the past two months, or the physician does not have a sound rationale for re–ordering it.
2. The Drug is stopped or dosage decreased for a period of four to eight weeks (depending on the half life of the specific medication).

3. A back–up prn sedative is ordered in case the behaviour returns during the trial period and threatens to become uncontrollable.
4. All staff are required to report and record behavioural and/or functional changes noted during this time, whether better or worse.
5. If the originating behaviour does not recur during the trial period, the back–up prn sedative is discontinued, the original drug is stopped, or in the case where the dosage was lowered, it is lowered further.

THE 24 HOUR PROFILE

We have identified repeatedly to this point that the mentally impaired are vulnerable to a number of factors – the time of day, the stimuli around them, staff's approach, etc. This establishes some key factors that influence effective assessment:
   – No one staff member can know any one resident totally (what he is capable of doing, how he behaves, etc.) 24 hours per day, seven days a week.
   – No one staff member can know all of what the rest of the team does that is successful or creates problems with all residents on the unit each shift.

The 24 Hour Profile may be the key to ensuring that information is communicated to all.

The 24 Hour Profile Questionnaire

The intention of the following team assessment is to provide a profile of a specific resident's functioning level over a 24 hour period. The goal of this information is to:

1. Identify changes in functioning noticed between shifts (days, afternoons and nights).
2. Identify the resident's strengths and limitations.
3. Identify successful techniques or approaches employed by certain staff in each area.

(Note: Only the questionnaire section of the 24 Hour Profile is presented in these pages. The complete questionnaire is located in the appendix at the back of the book. What is missing is the space to check off "Yes" or "No" for each statement and the supportive data section that is completed by day, afternoon and night shift.)

Instructions

Step 1

This questionnaire is to be initiated by a staff member who best knows the resident to be assessed. That staff member is required to complete the Supportive Data section for the shift that she has most contact with this resident (day, evening or night shift). Be as specific as possible, recording any supportive data you believe appropriate to describe this individual's functioning in each area. In the space under Supportive Data include the following:
- pattern of behaviour (time of day, equipment to be set in a specific manner, specific items used, etc.).
- when have you seen changes (will or will not function)?
- what do you say or do to the resident to assist the person to function?
- have you found any effective means of encouraging the person to function?
- how can you tell if the individual is being pressured and it is best not to attempt the task at this time?

Step 2

The completed form is then reviewed by each shift (days, afternoons and evenings), adding to the information provided.

Step 3

Once completed, a list of care issues are extracted and the guidelines in resolving them outlined in the supportive data which provides the basis for the care plan.

ACTIVITIES OF DAILY LIVING
1) Mealtime
- needs assistance?
- easily distracted?
  (if yes, how is this dealt with)
- can only handle a few items at a time? (if yes, which & in what order)
- any special arrangement or items?

2) Hygiene
a) Bathing
- cooperative in tub? (if no, explain)
- needs assistance?
- any special arrangements or items?

b) Teeth/Hair
- needs assistance?
- requires articles to be handed to him/her?
- only requires articles be displayed?
- cooperative during procedure (if no explain)?
- any special arrangements or items?

c) Dressing
- requires assistance dressing or undressing?
- requires articles to be displayed?
- requires articles to be handed to him/her?
- problems with specific articles of clothing?
- can pick own clothing from closet?
- any special arrangements or items?

d) Toileting
- specific times? (which)
- needs to be checked? (when)
- how does he/she communicate the need to go to the washroom (does he tell you or by what actions)?
- any special arrangements or items?

3) Ambulation
- gait unsteady (describe gait)
- needs to be checked, will exhaust self? (what time of day and what is done if unsteady)
- wanders? (identify time and specific area)
- how do you deal with the wandering?

COMPREHENSION
- understands instructions? (if no explain)
- responds to his/her name? (first, last or nickname)
- can identify staff or family members? (who and how often)
- can identify all objects? (if no, what and when)

– finds way around unit? (room, washroom, dining room, lounge)
– what must you do to help this person understand what you are saying or what you want done?

BEHAVIOUR
In each area where (yes) is checked describe what the resident does and how you deal with it.
– restlessness
– repetitive behaviour
– destructive
– disturbing behaviour (who?)
– hoarding (what, from where?)
– verbally/physically threatening others

SOCIAL SKILLS
– can relate to others? (will talk to who, when and about what)
– helps others? (who & when)
– relates well to new people? (if no, explain what happens)
– participates in group activities? (what and when)

ACTIVITIES
– performs specific chores on the unit? (what and when)
– involved in specific games, hobbies? (what, when and for how long)
– reads or looks through books/magazines?
– enjoys music, TV (what and when?)

****

The completed form provides considerable insight into this resident's performance, needs and abilities. It also ensures that any approaches or procedures that a staff member may be employing with this resident is known by all.

A good example to demonstrate the benefits of this process involved a team discussion about a resident we will call Ann. This resident's cognitive ability was very limited, her attention span extremely short. The staff who initiated the form identified under "toileting" that she would always stand as soon as you sat her on the toilet causing her to be incontinent, urinating on the floor. All staff agreed with the problem, but no one voiced a solution until the afternoon conference reviewed the material. One of the part-time staff said she had worked out something that was effective even though it sounded kind of silly. She found if she sat Ann on the toilet, stood in front of her with her knees against her's and her face close to Ann's, that she would sit long enough to go. A simple solution to a complex problem.

The information received from the 24 Hour Profile provides the necessary direction for the care plan. After the profile has been reviewed by all three shifts, the information is compiled to identify the problems or issues encountered in providing care and the necessary approaches or interventions to be taken. The care plan now becomes a guide for any staff making contact with each resident.

THE INTERVIEW

Unfortunately, some do not use the interview in the assessment process. Considerable information can be gained from interviewing a mentally impaired resident. Through the interview, one can determine:

1. Attention Span
2. Emotional State
3. Language Pattern
4. Thought Process
5. Reminiscing ability
6. Set Precedent

A successful interview requires the interviewer to have established a degree of rapport with the resident. If on first contact one expects to obtain considerable accurate information, then the interviewer will be disappointed. The first contact with a resident is usually a situation where that person is meeting someone new. Answering questions for a person who is not familiar is anxiety producing. Being unable to answer some of those questions is even worse. By elevating the resident's anxiety, his mental functioning ability decreases and he is unable to concentrate or to think as clearly as under normal conditions. In that situation, it is not clear what the interviewer is assessing, the resident's actual functioning level or his anxiety level.

On the first interview the interviewer does not know how to adjust questions, posture and actions appropriately enough to be effective with this individual. It is important to know the resident before you can decide how to proceed.

Where you sit in relation to the resident is also crucial. In sitting directly beside him, you will become invisible (remember tunnel or narrowed vision – peripheral vision is lost) and interaction will be limited. Sitting directly in front of him is anxiety producing. He cannot look anywhere else but at you, which is too intense a stimulus, plus he will have the feeling of being closed in. The best location to sit is again at an angle to his dominant side. He can see you easily, but is also able to divert his eyes elsewhere if he becomes too stressed. That manner of posturing also leaves him an "escape route" if he finds his anxiety level increasing. In fact if that resident leaves after four minutes or four questions, do not be surprised. His leaving the interview is telling you his tolerance level, let him go and try again later. To force him to stay an additional fifteen minutes or for another fifteen questions, will result in creating an agitated resident. Remember to read the behavioural cues.

1. Attention span

The interview must be conducted in a quiet location, free from unnecessary noise and stimuli. The more familiar the environment to the resident the better (usually his room with the door closed). This ensures the resident is not distracted by other noise and movement. If the resident is unable to concentrate on what is being said, or to even sit longer than a few moments without getting restless, then that is a significant indication of the resident's attention span. If he is unable to concentrate on this very direct and intense stimuli, then he will have considerable difficulty lasting in any activity that is longer than a few moments. Defining the resident's attention span is important information for staff regarding the activities this resident is involved in – for this resident keep them "short and sweet".

2. Emotional state

It is important for the interviewer to uncover the emotional overtones of the resident's conversation. The emotional state of a mentally impaired resident can be expressed in many indirect ways. The resident talking about this place as a prison or the one who is suspicious during the interview provides considerable insight into the person's needs on the unit. If the individual's anxiety level is high, the emotions expressed will be ones of fear, requiring staff to invest considerable energy to establish rapport and security.

3. Language Pattern

The interviewer must be attentive, listening to the pattern of words during the conversation will give an indication of any language deficiencies. Using the word "brother" instead of "husband" may indicate that the person has forgotten her husband's name or her relationship to him and replaced it with the next nearest name – "brother". This process of replacing words is important to staff in determining effectively how to communicate with the resident, decreasing anxiety and stress.

4. Thought process

Some mentally impaired can experience disjointed thoughts, where each phrase expressed has no relationship to the other – "The moon is in the sky. I saw the chickens. Where's my daughter?" Staff encountering this resident may believe she is incapable of responding to any questions. It is important in the interview to determine if this resident is capable of responding appropriately to yes/no questions. If, in all of the rambling the resident does stop, respond appropriately to the question asked, and then continues rambling, staff must then be encouraged to ask short, concise questions on contact, such as "Do you need to go to the bathroom?" rather than assume she cannot respond.

5. Reminiscing

It is important during an interview not only to listen for the right answers to the questions being asked, but also to what the resident is talking about. Much of her conversation may be out of context to what is being discussed, but if you listen to what she is saying, it may make sense – she talks of her daughter when she was fourteen and is very accurate in her description of that past event. This lady becomes an excellent candidate for reminiscing. Staff can be instructed to carry on a conversation about her past and be fairly confident that the information she is sharing is accurate. Staff may also be successful in performing a process called progressive orientation – filling in the gaps, by talking to her about the time she believes it is, moving her forward to the present – "You daughter went to high school, didn't she? Then college . . . she got married . . . she has children. How old does that make you?"

6. Permission
What is more significant about having the interview as part of the assessment process is the permission it gives to staff – regardless of the mental functioning level of a resident, it is expected that staff will make one–to–one contact with that person. This fosters an understanding that a mentally impaired resident still needs to be heard and considerable information can be gained from what the resident says.

HISTORY

Family are the most important key for us to successfully care for the mentally impaired elderly. In fact, family members who have cared for their parent prior to admission are even more valuable. They may have already found what works and what causes problems concerning mother's care. Not to tap that information immediately means that staff will go through the same trial and error process, needlessly distressing the resident and being ineffective in their care.

Family can often help us fill in the "blanks" by not only giving us a clear picture of how they have cared for mother since she became impaired, but also of who mother was before the onset of the disease. A family questionnaire is essential. The questionnaire can be given to the family prior to, or on admission. They are asked to complete it to the best of their ability and then to review it with staff, to add any further details or complete areas that were unclear. That questionnaire must include the following:

Meals:
Likes and dislikes?
What will he eat if he refuses everything else?
What will he never eat?
When is his main meal?
What are normal meal times?
How much does he eat at each meal?
What problems have you had getting him to eat?
Any special arrangements or utensils used during meal time?

Does he snack during the day (if yes, what)?

Dressing:
What can he do for himself regarding dressing and
undressing?
What does he need help with?
Do you have any problems dressing or undressing him
(if yes, what and how do you deal with it)?
Is there anything he enjoys wearing more than others?

Toileting:
How do you know when he has to go to the bathroom?
Is he incontinent?
– if so, is he cooperative when you change him?
Is there a pattern, special times or manner that helps
you deal with toileting?
Are there any medication or foods taken to assist with
his bowels?

Bathing:
Does he normally have a bath or shower?
What time of day?
Any problems in bathing?
Special precautions or arrangements?
Would you be willing to be present during your
Mom/Dad's first bath or two after admission?
Problems combing and washing hair?
Problems with mouth care?
Does he brush his own teeth or do you do it for him?

Ambulation:
Does he wander?
– if yes, when and how long?
Is there a time of the day when you need to have him sit
so he does not become over tired?
What type of shoe does he wear?
Does he use any walking aids – cane, railing, walker,
etc.?

Activities:
What activities have you found he enjoys now?

What activities did he do in the past that he no longer
     does?
How long can he participate at an activity?
What is the best time for him to do activities?
Do you take him on outings?
     – if yes, where, when and how long?
What do you talk about?
Does he watch TV or listen to music?
     – if yes what type?
How often do you plan to visit?
Who plans to visit?
Are you willing to assist with activities or outings?
     – if yes, which day and time is most
     convenient?

Sleeping:
What time does he go to bed?
Is he up during the night (how often)?
Does he sleep during the day (when & how long)?
Anything special about his bed or room (personal quilt,
     number of pillows, light on, etc.)?
When he wakens at night how is his mental state?

Normal Day:
Describe a normal day for your dad.
When are his "bad times"?
How do you deal with those times?
When would we know he is getting anxious or agitated?
Do you have any problems getting him to take his
     medication?
Any special preparations for taking medications?
What things does he find comforting?
Is there a time of day that seems worse?
How does he relate to new people?

Understanding Your Mom/Dad:
Describe your Mom/Dad to me 20 years ago.
How has he dealt with stress all of his life?
What event(s) stand out in his life?

Once the information is obtained it is shared with the team
and incorporated into the care plan.

SUMMARY

The more we can understand who that resident was before the onset of the disease and what has occurred prior to admission, the better equipped we will be in establishing an environment specific to the needs of that person.

Assessment is an ongoing process. The emphasis begins from admission and is continuous for as long as we are caring for the resident. The challenge for the care team is to establish an assessment process that is both concise and effective, providing staff with a clear picture of the resident, his strengths and limitations, his needs and abilities. The more accurate our picture, the more effective our care.

Chapter Thirteen

Care Components

The basic concept in effectively caring for the mentally impaired elderly is to keep it simple. Simple, regarding what is expected for this person to remember and respond to. Simple, regarding what the person is asked to do and the instructions given. Simple regarding what you are able to do and how you do it.

ENSURING ACTIVITY INVOLVEMENT

When assessing a unit that houses a number of mentally impaired residents, I often ask recreation or activity staff to provide me with a list of the residents who fit the criteria for level two functioning ability. I then ask for a list identifying all of the activities they are involved in throughout the week. If programming for the mentally impaired is not an integral part of the care process and activity staff have not been encouraged to take an active role with this type of clientele, then I usually find that this group is often overlooked. Developing activities for those who are mentally impaired is challenging and requires considerable creativity and skill. Not all recreation staff are comfortable with this type of resident.

One way to ensure that the mentally impaired are not overlooked in activity programming is to specify the assignments of each activity staff member. This requires one person in the recreation department to be responsible for programming for those who are mentally impaired, and another responsible for activity programming for the physically disabled/cognitively well residents. This specifies the responsibility for researching and developing activity programming for each clientele.

Having specific activity staff accountable for a specific type of resident also ensures consistency at care conferences. Nursing staff know which recreation staff member should attend the care conference based on the functioning level of the resident discussed. In this way there is always the same activity staff member present who is best skilled in assessing that specific person's needs and determining which program is best suited.

Such a division in the recreation department does not imply that recreation staff work independent of each other. They are still expected to function as a cohesive department, assisting each other as needed in large group activities.

THE RANGE OF ACTIVITIES AVAILABLE

It is unfortunate that our industry has taken things of normal life and made them into therapies – music therapy, pet therapy, intergenerational programs. In some instances, that formalizing has decreased the spontaneity on the part of many staff, believing that it is not part of their role to be involved in such events. Activities are as significant in the life of a resident as bathing or eating. Quality of Life goes beyond the physical, requiring an investment of energy and resources in all parts of that person's life.

The list of activities available to the mentally impaired is endless. Nearly all activities appropriate for any older adult are appropriate for this clientele as long as they are adapted to the person's cognitive functioning level and physical and mental endurance capacity. Some of those activities include:

1. Communication groups

Communication groups of some type or another seem to be the trend now. Communication or discussion groups may be appropriate for the mentally impaired at level one of functioning. For many of the mentally impaired at level two, communicating for any length of time is a demanding process. To understand the pressure that communication groups can place on this individual, let us again compare it to the expectations placed on a person with right sided paralysis. If I were paralyzed on the right side of my body, you would not ask me to do things that required two hands. Instead, you would adapt the activity to match my limitations.

The same expectation must be true of the mentally impaired. Involvement in communication groups is totally dependent on the resident's ability. Most of the mentally impaired at level two of functioning will have difficulty with a group activity of this type.

In order to carry on a conversation a person must concentrate on what was just said, determine what needs to be said in reply and then decide where the conversation is leading – a process that the mentally impaired must find demanding and confusing. Most mentally impaired residents have difficulty carrying on a conversation with one person let alone a group of people. During a group discussion a mentally impaired resident is required to concentrate on one person speaking, try to understand what that person is saying and maintain the train of thought in order to reply. Suddenly another person speaks. Once again that resident must quickly identify who it is, concentrate on what is being said, then another speaks. The process repeats itself again and again.

During a group discussion, the mentally impaired are required to bounce from person–to–person in order to keep up with the conversation. To the mentally impaired this creates a state of bombarding – over stimulation that will result in the person feeling out of control, becoming increasingly agitated at the demands of the task or withdrawing from the stimulus experienced.

I have seen too many communication groups where the group leader (a staff member) talks to one resident, then moves to the next resident, with little or no interaction maintained between residents. The value of such an exercise is questioned. One might as well work with one resident at a time and forget the group rather than subject this type of resident to such a complex task.

This is not to say that communication groups should stop. With anything involving the mentally impaired – if it works, don't change it. Carrying on a conversation where you are the principal speaker and the resident is encouraged to participate when he wishes seems to be the least demanding for some. If the resident participates in any way, or is an active observer, then by all means continue with the group. If any resident merely sits there with little or no response, then that is not the activity for that person.

2. Sensory Stimulation

The most rewarding activities involving the mentally impaired are those that return to the resident the things that are normal to life.

A common experience of the mentally impaired in an institutional setting is sensory deprivation. You experience this state frequently yourself. How often at the end of your shift have you walked through the front doors of the facility and intentionally taken a deep breath of fresh air? That is a common response when one experiences sensory deprivation. Sensory deprivation occurs when the environment is void of the natural colours, aromas and sensations we are accustomed to experiencing.

The experience of sensory deprivation can be demonstrated with your residents as well. If the resident lounge in your facility is furnished with vinyl furniture, watch the response of a mentally impaired resident who has the opportunity to sit on a fabric covered couch. As soon as she makes contact with the fabric, she will continually stroke it. Her behaviour demonstrates the intensity of the sensation created by that material. She has not experienced such a sensation for a long time, and moving her hands over the cloth now, she finds it very intense and highly stimulating. The fabric creates sensory sensation. In fact many substances will create the same effect.

To re-create the effect, give a whole onion and a paring knife to a mentally impaired resident and then watch her response. She will act as though it were a major discovery. Encourage her to cut it, feel it and smell it and watch the reaction on her face. She may even take a bite from it – that will no doubt cause sensory stimulation.

When was the last time a mentally impaired resident has seen a caterpillar? In the spring I will search for a caterpillar and bring it into the unit. Making sure the resident is aware of what it is and it will not harm him, I will place it in his hand. The resident may squish it – sensory stimulation.

Spices, fabrics, sandpaper, anything that the resident has not handled for some time will have a phenomenal impact. Bring in a pile of leaves during the fall and just plop them on a table, or a bucket of snow in the winter and have residents place their hands in them. Their reaction will be most rewarding.

3. Music

Music to many older people means more than just entertainment. In fact, prior to the 1950's or the age of television, music was the main source of entertainment, encompassing almost every social event.

What was the top song in 1972?

I haven't the slightest idea. Ask an older person the top song during the war and he will probably be able to tell you. That song was heard thousands of times.

Play the "right" old song and certain mentally impaired residents who normally seem incapable of maintaining any conversation or coherent thought will sing that song from beginning to end without missing a word. That resident is probably singing from old memory, virtually back in the 1940's when she heard it so often.

Certain music brings back memories for all of us. A soft, conventional song can elicit a very positive response from many mentally impaired.

4. Children

Place a baby in the arms of a mentally impaired resident and you will probably see a dramatic shift in that person's behaviour. I remember when I was assessing one unit, a staff member brought in her newborn baby to show everyone. She approached a resident who had a history of aggressive outbursts. When one of the staff on duty saw what she was doing, she suggested that she not give the baby to "that" resident. I asked the mother how she felt about it. She responded "I think it will be okay as long as we watch." She handed the baby to this resident and the transition was almost instantaneous. The resident smiled, cuddled the baby and talked to it. Most of us learned to handle babies when we were children. It takes considerable memory loss to forget how to respond to a baby or a young child.

A number of facilities have implemented effective children's programs, formally called intergenerational programs. One such program is to have a child daycare centre within the facility. Few facilities have the resources to run one of these on their own. What they have done instead is to lease space within the facility to a privately run daycare business. In that way the operation of the daycare centre is not the responsibility of the facility, but the residents living in that facility are encouraged to participate through such avenues as the "hug–a–kid program". Many mentally impaired residents respond beautifully to such an opportunity.

Other facilities have linked resident programming opportunities with local schools, implementing an "adopt–a–grandparent program". This program encourages individual students or whole classrooms to adopt one resident as a "grandparent". The students are then encouraged to visit and send cards on special days. Whenever such a program is implemented, it is important that a representative of the facility present to the students information about the facility, the residents and their needs so that they are prepared for what they may encounter and what may be asked of them. Likewise, children involved with specific residents need to be buddied with a staff member or volunteer that knows the resident, who can act as a resource when the child visits.

Other "kid" programs involve older children who are encouraged to visit to help certain residents during mealtimes. In fact, many high schools have what are called life enrichment credits. These are recognized credited programs where students are allowed to take a certain amount of time each month from school in order to participate in a community based assignment. Assisting on specific units within a facility provides an ideal learning base for some students. Any of these programs are useful on any unit to establish an atmosphere that is normal and healthy.

By the way, the children are usually very receptive when involved with the mentally impaired elderly, as long as they are supported and prepared for what may occur on the unit. In fact the younger the child, the better the rapport. If any problems do occur, they usually arise from the parents. Stereotypic beliefs about a long term care facility and those who live within it may limit the open-mindedness of certain parents, which can make such opportunities for the children difficult. It is important before any program is implemented that the parents are helped to understand the purpose and role of the children's visits.

5. Pets

Many facilities have introduced pets to their units. Fish and birds are probably the most universal, dogs and cats are the up and coming rage. The pet used must be a "people sensitive animal", one that knows who and who not to go to. It must be remembered that there are many people who normally do not like cats or dogs. Likewise, there are certain mentally impaired residents who cannot tolerate them as well. To have a cat or dog jump without warning on the lap of such a resident will result in the cat or the resident being injured. The cat will be injured, when the resident grabs it to fling it off his lap. The resident will be injured, when he grabs the cat. If the animal cannot effectively determine which resident to avoid, then it should not be on the unit.

Some facilities have brought in dogs or cats from the local humane society. In some instances, this has created some difficulties. An animal that may appear friendly when in contact with one person may not be able to handle a unit with 30 people. One of the best animals to arrange for visitations are those from kennel clubs. These are well trained animals that the owners are pleased to display. Another source of pets for visitation is from staff themselves. Encouraging staff to bring in their own pets for the shift they are scheduled to work is very effective.

I always admire a facility that is willing to go "the extra mile" to provide to its residents the fullest degree of quality of life. One such facility had an enclosed courtyard. They would periodically put rabbits or a goat in that area. The residents would feed and talk to the animals. It was amazing to watch the response by some.

6. Bursts of Activity

As identified in our earlier discussion on wandering, it is not uncommon for the mentally impaired to have a poor attention span. Planned bursts of activity are important and must consciously be integrated into the care routine. If energy of the mentally impaired is not exhausted in a conscious effort, then it will impact on the success of any care task as the day progresses.

Activities such as turning on a radio and performing passive exercises with this resident, taking one arm and then the other and helping the person raise and lower them are simple interventions. Taking a resident or group of residents for a walk, going at a pace and distance that is within the person's physical limit is another quick option. Encouraging certain residents to follow staff as they conduct rounds or pick up equipment is always valuable. All of these simple activities are totally at the control of the staff responsible for those residents. When implemented on an ongoing and informal basis they not only release the built up energy of the resident, but also provide staff an opportunity to enhance their rapport with those under their care. By the way, the staff who work well with this type of clientele and who understand them, usually undertake such interventions if they are clear that they have the permission to do so.

7. Activities of Daily Living (ADL)

Integrating certain ADL tasks as programs is also valuable. An effective activity is to help a mentally impaired resident shave himself, who has in the past been shaved by staff. This simple task can accomplish a great deal more than mere shaving. Think about it for a moment! What needs to be done to help a resident shave himself? The steps would be as follows:

> Take the electric razor (turned off) and place it in his hand, then turn it on (sensory stimulation). With the resident sitting in front of the mirror and placing one hand on his shoulder and the other one guiding his hand with the razor, move the razor to his face identifying where on his face you are touching him and encouraging him to look in the mirror during the process.

What you have accomplished here is very meaningful. Sensory stimulation by feeling the razor on his own face and in his hand; sensory stimulation by touching him as you are doing the process; purposeful hand and arm movement, raising the razor to his face and moving it from one side to the other, a movement he may not have performed for some time; body awareness by identifying left and right side of his face, his chin, etc. There is a further side benefit to this task. If he is capable of performing this movement on his own, you can replace the razor with a face cloth or a spoon.

The important point in this activity is the following: whether he is capable of shaving himself or not, he is receiving the most beneficial commodity – your time and contact. A valuable activity.

8. Expanding Staff Contact

The following is a comment that usually raises some eyebrows – it is important that staff be allowed the freedom to stop at any time during their shift for a break or a cup of coffee, as long as they are having it with two residents who are mentally impaired. This becomes a rewarding program for both staff and the residents involved – an opportunity to spend time at a very simple task, but one that enhances rapport and improves communication. To provide this type of freedom requires an environment that trusts its staff. Such freedom is fraught with potential difficulties on some units that will be discussed in the next chapter.

One of the qualities demonstrated on the better units who care for the mentally impaired elderly is the ability to periodically do something a bit "crazy". No routine or schedule is set in stone. Staff need to be told that they can go anywhere they want during their work day, as long as they take their residents with them. This freedom to break the routine is an effective means to give staff the permission to be flexible. Taking the residents on a picnic or to the zoo provides an atmosphere of normalcy.

An integral and rewarding part of our job is to have "fun". If staff are enjoying themselves, the residents are probably having a good time as well.

9. Chores

Many of our residents will respond better to chores than to most recreational activities. Chores are tasks that the resident has performed all of his life. He may no longer be able to perform the task well or even to complete it, but he can still feel useful by attempting it.

When one remembers that our residents have been caregivers all of their lives, not care receivers, it is easy to identify how important chores become. There is a constant need for some mentally impaired residents to do what is familiar and what feels useful. It is not uncommon to see mentally impaired residents wiping table tops, picking up bits of paper or articles of clothing, even helping other residents. Their performance may not be complete or even accurate, but they are often focused on the task for a varying amount of time.

Chores must be integrated into programming. Washing 10 medicine cups over and over again, folding a couple of towels, cleaning table tops repeatedly, pushing a broom around, sweeping the same piece of dirt, all have a function. It is you who is aware of the task being repetitive, not the resident. If a mentally impaired resident was aware that he was completing the same task again and again, it would increase his anxiety and lead to an agitated response. Those who proclaim that a resident should not be allowed to do such a repetitive task because it is not normal, have forgotten that expecting "normal" behaviour is asking too much of our mentally impaired.

Once again, if I had right sided paralysis from a stroke and could only use my left arm, would you stop me from performing all tasks because I could not do them as a "normal" person? No, you would adjust the task to fit my existing strengths and limitations, praising me for performing at my best ability.

If I am mentally impaired, doing that one task over and over again may be my optimum functioning level. No one knows what doing that task means to me. It can provide a sense of purpose, a feeling of being needed, active range of motion exercises, energy release in a positive manner, etc. It is better to have a resident fold a couple of towels for a half an hour than stare at a blank wall for the same length of time or wander aimlessly through the hall.

There is an endless list of activities in which the mentally impaired can participate. To make any activity successful requires imagination and creativity. Again, "being a little crazy" is an important quality. To do things or try things that other staff may have trouble relating to, but are usually very effective, separates those staff who work well with the mentally impaired from those who do not.

ACTIVITIES – WHOSE RESPONSIBILITY?

Activities cannot be the responsibility of a single person or a single department. To believe that activity staff alone can spend the necessary time and energy with all mentally impaired residents, when their work ratio may be 50 to 1 (one activity staff to 50 or more residents) is totally unrealistic. To expect a mentally impaired resident to be able to respond to the same activity at the same time each day or each week is also unrealistic.

Beware of structure. Activities can be as ingrained as bathing, mealtime or bedtime. If a mentally impaired resident has had a bad night, where staff had to constantly struggle with him to get him up and then work diligently to settle him at the breakfast table, then why are they pushing him to his scheduled activity program at 0915 hours? Yesterday he may have successfully participated in that program. Today he will be unable to take part. In fact the activity program will probably only increase his agitation. Nursing staff must work together continually with recreation staff, communicating what is occurring as the resident is moved from one location to another or from one task to another. Any lack of communication will make it difficult for either staff to be successful and will only increase the stress experienced by the resident.

Breaking the barriers between departments is no easy task (see The Nurse Manager (& Others Too) in Long Term Care). Activities need to be integrated into the care process, making them the responsibility of each team member. In fact, the best time for some residents to get involved in an activity may be at 2:00 in the morning, when the person is up, wandering and has the potential of disturbing other residents. The effectiveness of integrating activity staff and their role with nursing staff and their responsibilities is very dependent on the cohesiveness of the care team. If the team is not functioning then effective resident care is impeded.

Activity staff must be encouraged to use their skills wisely. They have the expertise to determine the most appropriate activity a resident should be involved in, assessing how long that person can tolerate a specific task, the best time to run the activity, what to say to get the person motivated, how best to give instructions, what to expect, etc. Once this is discovered and an appropriate activity or set of activities is found, then that information needs to be given to the care staff. This provides all involved in a resident's day the needed information on what to do when spending time with this person, allowing activities to run when needed, not just when scheduled.

DEALING WITH REPETITIVE ACTIVITIES

Bob was a mentally impaired resident living in a LTC facility. Through the day, whenever he could find a napkin he would crunch it up and wander about the unit cleaning every table top he could find.

George is 78 years old, mentally impaired, living in a LTC facility. George ran a textile factory for forty years, where he mainly employed female employees. Now when George wandered the unit, if he found a female resident also wandering, he would take her by the arm and state "You are out of your work station dear" and proceed to take her back to her chair in the lounge.

251

In each of these cases, both men are simply demonstrating "old" behaviours. As stated earlier, the more you can understand the history of a mentally impaired resident, the better you may understand the person's present behaviour.

Talking with Bob's daughter-in-law, I asked her if there was anything in his past that she believed contributed to Bob constantly cleaning table tops. She said she couldn't think of a thing. Family are often not able to piece together what has happened in the past to what is being demonstrated now. They are just too close to the problem for that type of objectivity. I then asked her what significant events stood out for her in Bob's past.

She told me that just before she was about to marry Bob's son, her mother-in-law to be had a stroke. Bob was in a crisis. He did not want to institutionalize his young wife; he could not afford to quit work to take care of her; he could not afford to hire someone to stay with her five days a week. His only solution was to ask his daughter-in-law to be and his son to live in his home when they got married. Bob and his son would go to work and his daughter-in-law would take care of his wife.

You can imagine how difficult it must have been to ask his son and his new bride to do that. So he made a pact with his daughter-in-law. He told her "All I want you to do is take care of mother. Have supper ready for me when I get home, then get out of here. I will take care of the dishes, the cleaning, the dusting, the vacuuming, etc." This was his only way to compensate for the feelings he had in that situation.

He is doing now what he has done for thirty five years – clean. To him it has purpose. It is an activity that he can relate to. Unfortunately Bob's behaviour of cleaning table tops created one problem on the unit. It resulted in his cleaning any table he could find, including those in other resident's rooms. He would knock off the table anything that was in his way. This resulted in a few complaints by other residents and a number of complaints by staff to Bob's actions. The staff then tried to stop Bob's behaviour. Impossible! The only way to stop Bob was to sedate him or restrain im to a chair. Neither of those interventions were desirable. The only option left to staff was to make Bob's behaviour tolerable.

Rather than focusing on the areas that created difficulties (his limitations), they need to identify an area where he could clean (working with his strength). That area became the dining room. Staff were instructed that whenever they found him cleaning in a resident's room, they were to take him to the dining room, and encourage him to clean those tables as much as desired. The hope was that Bob would spend most of his cleaning time in the dining room. Please note the word "most". Staff knew that they could not be successful in stopping him 100% of the time from being in other resident's rooms, but at least now they had a specific intervention that was positive and supportive and his time was spent more in the dining room than anywhere else. His behaviour now became tolerable to all concerned.

In the case of George who escorted the ladies to their chairs, staff attempted to correct George, to no avail. As soon as staff saw him directing a resident to the lounge, they would say to him "George, this is a long term care facility. This lady is a resident. She lives here, she does not work for you. You don't have to take her to the lounge." George would respond "Thank you very much", then turn to the next female resident he saw wandering the hall and state "I am sorry dear, you are out of your work station" and proceed to accompany her to the lounge.

It is important to emphasize that you cannot stop the repetitive behaviour of the mentally impaired, all you can do is make it tolerable. You would wonder why staff would be concerned about George accompanying the ladies to the lounge. In fact on this unit wandering was almost non-existent with George around and one would almost think some of the ladies got up only to have George take them by the arm back to their chair. Problems arose from only one source. On this unit there lived a female resident who had the diagnosis of paranoid schizophrenia (suspicious of everyone around her). One thing you do not do with a paranoid schizophrenic is put your arms around her. Whenever George approached her a battle would ensue.

The only intervention left to staff was to ensure that whenever anyone saw George coming up the unit and the lady who was a paranoid schizophrenic going down, they had to separate them. That did not mean that staff would always be successful. It would be inevitable that at some time the two would meet and a battle would arise. All they could do was to make the behaviour as tolerable as possible.

In working with the mentally impaired, the best course of action is to determine what part of the behaviour creates the greatest difficulty and attempt to deal with that rather than to attempt to shut down the behaviour completely. Unfortunately some staff believe that the behaviour demonstrated by a specific resident is within that person's control. They regrettably believe that the mentally impaired have the ability to stop when told to. Nothing is further from the truth. The resident is acting the way he is because of the brain damage experienced. There is no way to reverse the damage, there is no way to stop the symptoms. Our responsibility is to make the behaviour tolerable. This requires considerable creativity for staff to determine how to channel repetitive behaviour to a more functional use – having Bob clean dining room tables; having George assist other residents to the lounge, etc.

As we delve further into the world of the mentally impaired we are demonstrating more and more the qualities of the effective staff member. It cannot be disputed that the staff member who invests this amount of energy into a person's care is a "special" person.

WHEN TO INTERVENE

We discussed under the section on chores the resident who performs the same activity again and again. This needs to be expanded in order to establish the premise for when to intervene on the activities of the mentally impaired.

> I am a mentally impaired resident, if I can get a towel, I will fold it, unfold it, fold it, unfold it, . . .

Are there problems with this behaviour? On the contrary, as discussed earlier, this activity may accomplish for this resident a great deal – provide a sense of purpose or feeling of being needed, constructively occupies time and releases energy, etc. Having the resident fold a towel for 20 minutes is better than staring at a blank wall for the same length of time.

Change the scenario slightly.

> I fold the towel, **I UNFOLD IT, I FOLD THE TOWEL AGAIN, U N F O L D I T,** . . . Each time I do it, I get more and more agitated.

254

Possibly, the resident in this situation believes she knows how she wants it completed, but she cannot get it to come out right or as she thinks it should be. The longer she is allowed to fold that towel, the more agitated she becomes. In this case the consequences of her having a towel to fold are negative. Therefore, you do not want this person to have a towel.

Intervention on repetitive activities of the mentally impaired is simply based on consequences – if there are no obvious negative consequences, then investing energy to stop that activity is a waste of time. If negative consequences are obvious, then it is important to intervene.

Whether the activity is considered normal or not is not the issue. Even though our responsibility is to treat that person as a normal adult, expecting a mentally impaired resident to perform any task "normally" is expecting too much. Our responsibility with the mentally impaired is not to demand from that person normal behaviour, but to prevent further impairment or dysfunctioning. Intervening in areas that demonstrate negative consequences is intended to enhance the person's well being, maintain safety and improve his quality of life.

Any behaviour of a mentally impaired resident can be examined in this manner.

> A 76 year old lady was admitted to a LTC facility and during her first three months on the unit she continually clutched an empty record album cover to her chest. The album cover had a face on it and she attempted to have it with her all of the time.

Do you see a problem with this behaviour? In the short term "no", over the long term – "yes". It is important to re–emphasize that this lady was only admitted to the unit three months before. The anxiety from the transition shock of admission may still be fairly intense. Familiarity to the unit even after three months may not yet be established. This lady is communicating her anxiety and her needs directly to us by her actions – her hugging an inanimate object demonstrates her feelings of insecurity. This is not unusual behaviour. We all become attached to inanimate objects.

Do you have your chair in your home? One in which your family knows that you will always sit. What happens as soon as you are in that chair? You relax! That chair provides you with a sense of security. There is no difference in your response to your chair than this lady to her record album. The album provides the security she needs in order to cope with the pressures of living on the unit. Again the obvious immediate consequences are not negative. In fact this is an important support for this lady that allows her to cope with the stresses experienced on the unit.

Some staff where this resident lived felt that her reliance on the album was not an immediate problem that needed intervention. They felt that if it was important for her to hold onto the album at this time, then they should let her have it. Other staff saw it differently. They said "It is not normal behaviour, take it away from her." It is terrible being confused in a confusing environment. Some shifts she was allowed to have the album, other shifts it was yanked away from her. The lack of consistency by the staff only intensified this lady's frustration and inability to cope with living on the unit.

In the short run, her need to hold onto this album was not a problem. In the long run, it had the potential of becoming a serious problem. Imagine the effects upon this lady if she was required to focus on this inanimate object as her only means of security for an entire year. Eventually she would demonstrate some very bizarre behaviour as a result. It is our responsibility to always remember that the behaviour of the mentally impaired will always communicate their need. To ignore what is observed and leave a mentally impaired resident to solve her own problem will always result in the response being inappropriate.

The responsibility of the staff was to replace this inanimate object with something animate. In this case, three staff were assigned to this lady, where each staff member was on opposing shifts to the other two (days, evenings and nights). This ensured that at least one of these staff were on duty through most of the week. Each of the staff assigned to her, were instructed to be involved in her care as much as possible over the next three months. If they could not be assigned directly to her on certain shifts, then they were required to start and end their shift by making contact with her – saying hello, finding out how she was, spending a few moments with her. The goal was to increase familiarity. Hopefully the resident would be able to recall some or all of the staff by face alone, allowing the development of a strong rapport between those staff and herself. Even if she could not remember any of the staff by face, at least the repeated contact would allow the staff to determine the most effective approach and care tactics specific to this lady. This would allow them to identify the best ways to provide a secure environment on each shift. As the next three months passed, the staff were to wean the resident from the album or at least provide for her other avenues of gaining security other than the album itself. Slowly they would be shifting her focus from the inanimate object (the album) to something animate (the staff).

The need to intervene on the behaviours of the mentally impaired is totally dependent on the consequences experienced. If there are very obvious negative consequences, then it is important to intervene. If not, then there is no problem.

Let us change the scenario. Instead of this resident responding to the album as she did, imagine her reacting in the following way:

> She talks to the face on the album. If you talk to her, she does not respond. If someone tries to take the album from her, she will become aggressive.

The negative consequences are obvious:

> 1. The stimuli is too intense − the face on the album is too closely linked with her reality and she cannot separate it from what is real and what is not, drawing her further and further from the "here and now". This will eventually result in her functioning ability deteriorating over time, losing further contact with what is happening about her.

> 2. The album is so intense it decreases her interaction with those around her.

> 3. The potential for an aggressive outburst when the album is taken from her is high.

This lady requires the same opportunity to gain security with staff as described above, but her having an album would have very negative consequences.

This is an important concept when considering interventions with the mentally impaired. To differentiate the necessity between consequences, recall the mirror. We discussed that some mentally impaired residents become very agitated when looking into the mirror. Those who believe they are 45 years old, suddenly see the reflection of an 85 year old man. The reality shock experienced when they know it is their reflection will result in severe agitated response. The obvious intervention is to remove mirrors from this resident's view (especially in his room and bathroom). The goal for such an intervention is to prevent the negative consequences created by the stimulus. Likewise, it is important to remove the record album from the resident who is incapable of coping with it. The stimuli is too intense, impairing her ability to function effectively. The same premise is true with all aspects that involve the mentally impaired. When the consequences are negative we must intervene for the sake of the resident. The foundation of Quality of Life, the goal of Supportive Therapy.

THE DOLL

Let us continue with the mirror relationship. We identified that some mentally impaired residents who see their reflection in the mirror haven't the ability to know it is themselves. As a result, they talk to the mirror possibly believing that it is someone standing on the other side of a window. When that occurs, no one would be heartless enough to say to that resident "Let's talk to that person in the mirror." All would agree that such a response would be totally inappropriate.

This leads us to a popular question I am frequently asked – should a mentally impaired resident be given a doll? As always there is no simple answer, it depends on the circumstances. If the resident's response to the doll is that she wants it in view, always with her, then there is no obvious negative consequences. Therefore let her have it.

On the other hand, if the resident talks to the doll, cradles it, tries to feed it and dress it, will not talk to anyone else because she is so engrossed with the doll and will become agitated if you try to take it away from her, then that is a different story.

A doll lies! It is the size of a baby, it looks like a baby, is the colour, shape and feel of a baby. It is so close to reality, that it may be too difficult for a mentally impaired resident to differentiate it from the real thing. Besides, how do others talk about the doll to the resident? When this lady says "get my baby", what do staff bring her?

If I said to you, "Do you see the chickens under the table?", would you respond "Yes Len, I'll put them in the barnyard for you." Lying to a mentally impaired resident only reinforces that person's reality as accurate – causing major problems in this resident's functioning ability. Reinforcing for this resident that the doll is a baby is no different than putting the chickens in the barn or carrying on a conversation with the reflection in the mirror. In each case the response is inappropriate.

The doll for some staff is an easy solution. Their rationale is "It keeps her quiet, let her have it." If that is the reason for her having the doll, then the staff involved have not looked closely enough at the consequences and what this resident may be communicating.

Our residents have been caregivers all of their lives, not care receivers. Being mentally impaired does not mean that there is no longer a need for a purpose, or more importantly, a need to be needed. If I can't find someone who needs me, I will find something.

The resident who must talk to and feed a doll, needs the doll replaced with a real baby or young child. Allowing this resident the opportunity to have contact with a child may meet a very significant, deep seated need to nurture. In fact this is the resident who can best benefit from contact with the facility pet, allowing her to care for and hold the cat or dog. At least a child or an animal are more rational ways of meeting a person's need.

More importantly, you can "give me you"! It is common for many of our residents to experience the ultimate in sensory deprivation – touch. How often is a mentally impaired resident in a long term care facility held? Probably quite infrequent, if at all. All of us know what it is like to be depressed or scared. As those feelings intensify, so does our need to be held. Physical contact is a way to feel secure, a way to be comforted through the stress experienced. When there is no one there to provide such a support, there will always be something. In the case of the mentally impaired resident, it can easily become the doll.

Certain staff are not comfortable touching residents other than during care – bathing or dressing. Those staff find it difficult to approach a resident sitting in a chair and place their hands on his shoulders for longer than a few moments. To have to hug a resident would be very uncomfortable, and with some totally impossible. That's fine! Staff should feel free to admit their own limitations. Not all of us have the same comfort zones and abilities.

259

On the other hand, there are staff who are the complete opposite. They enjoy putting their arms around a resident, hugging and holding them whenever it is needed. We need to know who those staff are and encourage them to do it more. Every care team must tap the strengths of each of its members and utilize those strengths with the most appropriate resident to ensure effective caring. Good physical care is only one part of our job. Being supportive involves every aspect of the resident's world.

I am not suggesting that we rip the doll away from a resident who has had one for years. As I did not suggest that we take the record album from the individual who used it in order to cope. Our responsibility is to replace that doll with what is needed – a purpose, touch and a supportive care setting.

That also means that we talk about issues as they exist, not as the resident perceives them. We know the perceptions of the mentally impaired resident will always be inaccurate. As we would not confuse them further by talking to the reflection in the mirror, we cannot talk to the resident as those the doll is a baby. When the resident asks for her baby, the staff's response must be "I will bring your doll to you." You may consider that a subtle difference, but it is the difference that matters in caring for the mentally impaired.

There is one more reason why providing a doll to a mentally impaired resident is inappropriate. It relates to an earlier point made when discussing those just developing the disease. If you remember, I shared with you a common fear of those at level one of functioning – "The disease is one thing that scares me. What is just as frightening is to know that soon I will lose control over my own dignity and will rely totally on others to control it for me."

Without intervention, the doll has the ability to elicit from a mentally impaired resident a response that can be called "infantilism" – childlike behaviour. Make this personal. You walk onto the unit and see your 78 year old, mentally impaired mother on the floor playing with a doll. What would be your response? What has happened to her dignity? It takes more creativity and skill to replace that doll, than to just give it to her to be quiet.

I will allow nothing to divert me from fulfilling my vow to maintain the dignity of the mentally impaired under my care. That is the first and foremost in determining any intervention employed. It is the premise for the basic concept of Supportive

Therapy – "We treat the mentally impaired as though they are normal adults, but we do not expect normal behaviour."

WHAT TO SAY

Before discussing this topic, it is important to compare its length to the rest of the book. This section on what to say to the mentally impaired will only encompass a couple of pages. Our discussion on the other options of care required substantially more time and space.

A verbal response to a mentally impaired resident is of minimal significance for a number of reasons. First, the person's poor memory retention and comprehension skills makes what we say only a temporary intervention. Anything that is said to a mentally impaired resident is often forgotten as soon as it is heard. Secondly, we have already established that the world of the mentally impaired is very real to them. Continually contradicting or correcting, strips away from that resident what he believes is right and may create further confusion or even an agitated response.

It is more important that we invest our energies and resources into developing effective and flexible programming than to concentrate excess energy on the skill of what to say. It is the programming – the environment, the care routines, the approach, the concepts, etc. that will effect this resident more than anything else. If they are not adequately developed, nothing we say will have the least effect. Besides, there is no magic statement that will stop the repetitive demands or questions of the mentally impaired. If there were, I would have given it to you in the first few pages of this book. Knowing that there is no simple verbal response, the only approach that remains is to be supportive.

In order to respond to the question of what to say to a mentally impaired resident, we must return to the first chapter of this book. We began this text with a discussion about the importance of empathy – the ability to see the situation as the mentally impaired resident sees it. The more we can understand what the resident is experiencing, the more accurately we can adjust our approach or intervention.

Imagine:

> You have a personal problem/
> You come to me for counseling/
> I ask "What is your problem?"/
> You spend a few moments sharing it with me/
> I respond "Now that is the silliest thing I have ever heard
> I can't understand why you would get so upset about such
>   a simple thing as that."/

What just happened to our relationship? Would you talk to me again? Let us change that scenario slightly.

> You have a personal problem/
> You come to me for counselling
> I ask "What is your problem"/
> You spend a few moments sharing it with me/
> My response "That problem must be very important to you
> How can I help?"/

What just happened to our relationship? Would you talk to me again? This latter response enhanced rapport or trust between the two of us. In dealing with your problem, it is not important whether I agree or disagree with what is bothering you, instead it is my job to be supportive to help you deal with it.

Let us return to the case of "Marg" who we discussed in the chapter on aggression. If you remember, Marg always left the washroom after she was prepared for bed by pounding her fist and stating "They're stealing my clothes. They're stealing my clothes. They're . . ." The response by some staff when they met her in the hallway was "No one is stealing your clothes Marg."

If you can demonstrate that reality orientation works, then I say "go do it". Unfortunately, repeatedly correcting the mentally impaired does not change the resident's perception of what is happening. The impact of using reality orientation on every occasion can be compared to hitting the person over the head with a two-by-four or throwing a cold bucket of ice water at him. Bluntly correcting the resident with no sensitivity to what he is experiencing is in essence saying to the mentally impaired "You are wrong." That limited response only strips away the resident's reality (how he sees it), when he cannot relate to our reality (how we see it), therefore leaving him with nothing. His only response is to become more confused or agitated due to the intensified anxiety created.

In Marg's case, there is a more appropriate response:

> "Marg, if I believed someone was stealing my clothes, I'd be angry to. Let's sit down and have a cup of coffee."

While sitting and having a cup of coffee, we did not once talk about clothes. This approach simply distracted her from what she was looking for. The effect was to <u>temporarily</u> decrease her agitation and stop her repetition. It also enhanced my relationship with Marg by increasing our rapport. By being supportive she felt less threatened by me than the other staff who challenged her repeatedly. This was evident by the things I could get her to do that others were unsuccessful in achieving.

By the way, it is a mistake to believe that such a simple reply would completely stop Marg's calling out. As soon as she left the table and stepped into the hallway, she began again "They're stealing my clothes, . . ." If a simple verbal reply was all that was needed to stop her behaviour, then it wasn't Alzheimer's Disease that was causing it.

Staff like yourself who work "magic" – who are successful with certain mentally impaired residents when others are not – are successful because you take that person seriously. Regardless of the content of what the resident is saying, the emotions surrounding it are real. You cannot dissolve the emotions by just telling the person he is wrong.

Personalize what we are discussing. If you believed that someone had just stolen an article of your clothing, you would be upset. To tell you "No one has stolen your clothing", does not stop the anger you are experiencing. Nothing would satisfy you until you investigated for yourself whether it was gone or not. The same is true with the mentally impaired. Marg believed that someone stole her clothing. She was angry. Telling her she was wrong did nothing about the emotions she felt.

We have emphasized frequently throughout this text that there can never be only <u>one way</u> to deal with any behaviour of the mentally impaired elderly. There are no two residents who are the same, there can be no universal response to fit all. The same is true in what to say, staff cannot be limited to only one response. Diverting will work with some of the mentally impaired, but not with all. Staff cannot work from a "black/white" perspective, believing there is only one thing that can be done. They must be flexible to adjust to the specific needs of each resident. What must be used when communicating to the mentally impaired is a Supportive Approach, one that provides three possible responses:

If I believed _____, I would feel _____ as well,
then divert, correct or reminisce.

The first part of this response reinforces the empathy that has been emphasized throughout our discussion. "If I believed _____, I would feel _____ as well" requires us to put ourselves in the situation of that mentally impaired resident, to see the world as he sees it (personification). Once we understand the experience, we will know the emotions that are associated with it.

The second part of the response – divert, correct or reminisce provides options in how to respond. Diverting is an attempt to get the person's mind off of what he is looking for or what is disturbing him. This is an effective intervention at times. By steering him to something else he will forget what he was saying, only to return to it once the diversional activity is completed.

A second option is to correct. At times, giving a mentally impaired resident the information that is lacking may be appropriate. This manner corrects with a little more compassion. In Marg's case:

"Marg, if I believed someone was stealing my clothes, I'd be angry to, but your clothes were dirty and need to be washed. Let me take you to the dirty utility room and I will show you where they are."

A slight reminder or simple clarification for some mentally impaired is all that is needed. The resident may respond "Oh, that's nice, thank you." Only minutes later it will soon be forgotten and she will return to the hallway, pounding her fist stating "They are stealing my clothes, . . ."

The third option is to reminisce or talk about what the resident is saying. We often forget that we can still speak to a mentally impaired resident about the problem without having to correct the content.

Take another example to demonstrate how the Supportive Approach can be utilized. A resident says to you "My baby is hurt. My baby is hurt". Simply place yourself in that person's situation. Right now you believe something has just happened to one of your children, how would you feel? The response in return would be:

"If I believed something happened to my child,
I'd be worried too. . ."

You now have three possible responses that you can make to complete that sentence:

1. Divert – steer the resident to something that will temporarily get her mind off of "the baby".
2. Correct – "I can understand how you believe that there may be a baby crying, it is Mrs. Smith in the next room calling out, let me show you."
3. Reminisce – "your children must be very special to you, tell me about them."

The tactic you use depends on the resident and the time you have available. If correcting the resident creates further agitation or confusion, then divert or reminisce. If the resident is incapable of carrying on a conversation, then correcting or diverting become the only options. If the resident becomes agitated when diverted, then reminiscing or correcting become the avenues to take.

No matter what is said, that resident's concern, questions or needs will be expressed again and again (like a scratched record with the needle caught at the same place, replaying itself over and over again). The only salvation, if you consider it as that, is time. As the disease worsens, the memory or awareness of that event or issue will pass. All we can do in the interim is to be supportive, assisting the resident with what he is experiencing to the best of our ability.

UNDERSTANDING OUR LIMITS

A male mentally impaired resident
In his late seventies
Is living in your facility/

His wife died two years before admission/
When you sit him his table for a meal
He exclaims, "Set another place for my wife please, she
        will be here soon"/
Whenever you put him to bed he always asks,
"Would you leave the light on for my wife, she will be
        coming to bed soon?"/
Frequently when you meet him in the hall
He will stop you and ask, "Have you seen my wife, I think
        she has gone shopping?"/

While I was assessing this gentleman, he asked me "Would you like to meet my wife?" I responded "John, if I had not seen my wife for some time, I'd really miss her. The staff tell me your wife died two years ago." Tears came to his eyes. This man was not only impaired, he was grieving the loss of his wife.

The mentally impaired will recall memories that have attached to them intense emotions, either positive or negative. Each time the memory is recalled, those emotions will follow. Be comfortable with the emotions expressed by your mentally impaired residents, whether they evoke tears or anger. You will experience them frequently.

In fact family will often say to me – "I don't like talking to Dad about the past, I feel it will make him worse." They believe that because dad cries or gets angry, they have done something wrong. On the contrary, if you don't talk to him about his past, what else do you talk to him about? All he has left is the past.

In John's case, my next response was – "John tell me about your wife, she must have been an important part of your life." That response didn't resolve his emotions nor prevent him from asking about his wife only minutes later. It did allow him to talk about an important part of himself, a major component at that moment for his quality of life.

THE TABOOS OF "WHAT TO SAY"

There are two things that can be detrimental to the mentally impaired – to lie or to delve further.

Imagine, you have an 84 year old mentally impaired resident, who repeatedly asks "Where is my mother?". Some staff respond "Don't worry dear, your mother will be here in a half an hour." In actual fact, his mother died 30 years ago. If you asked those staff the reason for their lie, they will usually state "it 'is to keep her quiet". Generally, those are the same staff who will give the resident a doll, sedate or restrain that person, in order to accomplish that one, primary mandate – keep him quiet.

Lying reinforces the resident's perception of reality. Those who think it is the best intervention have not looked closely enough at the potential long term consequences. Such a response may quiet the resident temporarily. Over the long term it could create more difficult problems to resolve. Reinforcing that resident's reality will only intensify his past orientation, increasing his confusion. You have conditioned the resident to focus on something that he can easily recall. He will go from asking once every hour, to every five minutes.

The other taboo in communicating with the mentally impaired is to delve further (unfortunately this is becoming a popular trend employed by some). Delving further into what a mentally impaired resident says is the same principle employed while counselling. The counselors responsibility is to uncover the client's problem. To accomplish that goal, the client is forced to define or detail every word or statement. The more details that are added, the better the problem will be understood. Let me demonstrate.

Imagine:
> You are cognitively well
> You feel your world is "closing in on you" /
> The stress and emotional pressure you are experiencing
> Makes you feel as though you are out of control/
> You come to me for counseling/
>
> I ask "What is your problem?"
> You respond "I really don't know what it is.
> All I know is that nothing is going right."/
> "What do you mean `nothing is right'?"
> "My husband is driving me crazy"
> "What is it about your husband that effects you that way?"
>
> With each statement you make
> You are required to provide specifics/
> The problem will eventually be uncovered/
> At that moment

You will experience intense emotions
Either anger or tears/
Once those emotions are expressed
I can then help you
To learn how to solve your problem/

There is a new and popular technique that professes to be an effective way to converse with the mentally impaired elderly. It encourages making the mentally impaired define every word and phrase in order to uncover the true meaning of what the resident is saying. The goal is to uncover the real problem. There is no question that a mentally impaired resident may be able to respond to that mode of questioning. It is very likely that the conversation would focus the resident more on what is bothering him. It is also likely that when that problem is detailed further, you will also stir within that resident very intense emotions, either anger or tears. Now what do you do?

You cannot teach this individual how to resolve what is bothering him. He will forget any instructions or skills you give him. What is more important is the residual impact of such an approach. When you leave, he will have forgotten what was discussed, but will retain the emotions stirred. What has been the benefit of the time and energy invested? Such an approach is often fruitless and stacked with potential problems.

Staff will ask "How do you deal with a resident who continually asks `Where is my mother?', when you are in her room doing her care for 20 minutes?" The best response:

"If I hadn't seen my mother for a long time, I would really miss her. What did your mother do? What did she like to wear? What was she like?"

I would rather have that resident talk to me about her mother (reminisce) than ask continually where her mother is. There is no need to go any deeper in discussing the feelings she is experiencing by the loss of her mother, it will not help. Just carry on a normal conversation as you would with anyone else who was interested in talking about her mother. The only difference in the conversation between the resident and yourself is the grammatical tense that is used. The resident will talk in the present tense, you need to talk in the past tense. When the resident says "I would like you to meet my mother." Your response should be "I wish I could have met your mom, I bet she was a very nice person." Again it is subtle, but to argue will only create agitation, to go any deeper will create distress and to lie will only cause further confusion. What is left is to be supportive.

SUMMARY

Do not look for simple answers when caring for the mentally impaired. There are none. If there were, the family of our mentally impaired residents would have found them long ago and still be caring for their parent at home.

There are no "black/white, this/that" answers. For some who would like things neatly packaged that is frustrating, they see the challenges presented by the mentally impaired as problems that must be resolved, not realities that they must learn to live with. In fact those are often the staff who have the greatest difficulty with this clientele.

Others find the challenges created by the mentally impaired as exciting. They know that with this clientele you need to constantly be thinking, constantly creative, and fully involved in what you do. Those who thrive on "the challenge" are the ones who provide to this clientele the greatest level of quality of life possible, given their limitations and strengths. Those staff are always impressive to watch in action.

Regardless of the staff member, there is one fact that remains – to be effective, staff require a supportive work setting. Such a setting must encourage flexibility and creativity. It must support those staff who are successful with the mentally impaired and instill in others the same drive and insights.

Chapter Fourteen

Staff and Family

There is no cookbook or magic formula when caring for the mentally impaired elderly. Each staff member must determine on every contact what is needed and how it must be satisfied with every mentally impaired resident. This book has emphasized that successful caring of the mentally impaired is dependent on how staff perform that care. Those staff who are successful, possess some very unique qualities. They must be:

Part Elephant
Part Duck
Eyes of a Hawk
Patience of a Saint
Rationality of Mr. Spock
Personality of Mother Theresa

In fact if you were to combine these qualities into one picture, the <u>perfect</u> staff must look like this:

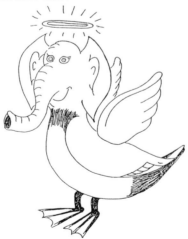

[My appreciation goes out to the family member of an Alzheimer's victim who diligently worked to create this caricature.]

Even though comical, it is a very accurate description of those staff who are successful with the mentally impaired. The qualities represent:

1. Part Elephant

Staff must be "thick skinned". At times staff can encounter both verbal or physical outbursts from some mentally impaired residents. Staff must understand that the resident's behaviour is related to his impairment, and often his comments or reactions has little to do with the staff member as an individual. To be "thick skinned" is to be able to experience these outbursts and not have it effect their relationship with the resident.

2. Part Duck

There are days that staff will struggle with a resident just to do basic care. Days where relating to this person is in itself the greatest challenge, stretching patience to its limit. It is the next contact or the next day where staff need to have virtually forgotten what happened and start fresh, letting things "roll off their backs".

3. Patience of a Saint

To get certain residents to perform tasks or to understand what is required takes time, perseverance and patience.

4. Eyes of a Hawk

Assessing a mentally impaired resident requires staff to see things that are not easily visible to others. Staff's vision or insights must be acute, constantly looking for the problem and adjusting their approach based on what is found.

5. Rationality of Mr. Spock

At times staff need to be totally objective and rational, times where they just need to "do". If a resident is soiled and refuses to be cleaned, and no persuading, no cajoling seems to be effective, the reality is that the job has to be done now or it will never be done – objective, rational approach with considerable tact like Mr. Spock from the movie Star Trek.

6. Personality of Sister Theresa

Staff require the compassion of Sister Theresa.

These descriptions provide a profile of our best staff members – those who possess the greatest amount of caring and compassion in dealing with this clientele mixed with considerable knowledge and skills. Yet no staff can effectively care for the mentally impaired unless the needed supports are in place. A philosophy that has is true in any work setting:

> The level of care staff provide to the resident is totally reflected by how well the facility takes care of its staff. (This has little to do with money.)

It is not possible in long term care to constantly supervise staff. Given the nature of the job and the limited number of management personnel, staff must be self–managers. No one knows what a staff member does in a resident's room when the door is closed.

The initiative for almost everything discussed must come totally from the individual doing the care. Maintaining that initiative places incredible demands on the caregiver. If the needed supports to perform the job are not in place and working well, staff enthusiasm to do their best will be lost over time. Once staff morale drops, so does the quality of care.

Staff require three supports to effectively care for the mentally impaired resident (or any resident for that matter):

Permission
Accountability
Recognition

PERMISSION

Giving staff permission allows them to freely adjust routines and care based on what is needed. Baths being done at a specific time, beds completed by 10 am, all residents in the dining room at a specific time, all meals must be completed within a half an hour of serving, and so on can create nothing but chaos in dealing with the mentally impaired. Allowing staff the permission to do their job, virtually allows staff to be flexible, to adjust their day to meet the needs of that resident at that time.

Flexibility requires trust. Trusting staff will do the job they were hired to do. This freedom provides staff with many options. One is to allow staff to have a coffee or a break whenever they want, as long as they are having it with two mentally impaired residents. As discussed earlier, this is a meaningful program in that it allows staff and residents to socialize. Such freedom indicates to staff that they can be trusted to do their job and stop when they need to, not just because it is break time.

It is interesting that every staff member every morning in every long term care facility requires his/her coffee break at the exact time – 10 am. Almost all facilities routinely have their break at that time. In working with the mentally impaired, a break is needed when a break is needed. If the routine is so structured that the break must be taken at 10 am, then all tasks are focused around that time regardless of the resident's functioning ability.

Permission includes allowing staff to enjoy themselves in their jobs. Having fun in this profession is essential, not just for the staff but for the residents as well. If taken too seriously, this job can exhaust anyone. Humour becomes a way to survive that which can be a very tedious, repetitive and emotionally draining job.

ACCOUNTABILITY

If staff are given the permission to do their job, then they are also accountable for what they do.

No matter how good a facility is, there are always a small percentage of staff who can be called "negative". The motives of these staff to work in a long term care facility are suspect. If a person is not working for the resident's sake, then he/she is simply there for a pay cheque. This is the staff person who is very structured in his or her routine, getting the job done regardless of the resident's need at any specific time. Interestingly enough, it is this staff member who will want to care for the mentally impaired, rather than the cognitively well when there is <u>no</u> programming, or the programming is not <u>enforced</u>.

> If I am mentally impaired and a staff member brings me breakfast, but doesn't give it to me for 20 minutes, would I know the difference?

> If you are cognitively well, physically disabled and that same staff member brings you breakfast and the coffee is cold, will she hear about it?

> If I am mentally impaired and my bath is normally at 0800 hours and the same staff member does it at 0600 hours, would I know the difference?

> If you are cognitively well, physically disabled and your bath is normally at 0800 hours and that staff member tries to do it at 0740, will she hear about it?

If there is no clear–cut programming for the mentally, impaired or programming is not enforced, then the "negative" staff will gravitate to the mentally impaired for the simple reason that this group can be so easily manipulated into any routine the staff desires. This staff member has the greatest difficulty with the aggressive mentally impaired and more often than not may be the primary cause of much of that person's aggressive behaviour.

Accountability sets an expectation that when something is to be followed through by staff, it is. When not followed through and insufficient reason is given, then that staff member must be answerable.

If staff are not made accountable, then there is no team. If any one team member is allowed to do what he/she wants, regardless of the team's direction, then the team is severely weakened. All decisions made in care will be frequently overturned by specific staff. Those staff who are motivated to provide the greatest level of quality of care will eventually feel as though they are always going "four steps ahead, and three steps back". They start something with a resident, just to find when they return after being off duty, it has not been followed through by other staff. If staff are not made accountable or answerable for their actions, then the team's motivation and enthusiasm will eventually wane and the quality of care will diminish as well.

Any lack of consistency on the part of staff creates a confusing environment for the resident. As well, it turns a 24 hour day into three eight hour periods, where every shift something different is expected and done. That confusion can only intensify a mentally impaired resident's anxiety level, resulting in chronic agitated behaviour, further impairing that person's ability to function.

RECOGNITION

If a mentally impaired resident on admission is aggressive and frequently attempts to leave the building, and then after 6 months on the unit the resident is no longer aggressive, no longer attempting to leave the building, not sedated and not restrained, what happened?

The staff did a good job. They set up the care and environment in a manner that provided for that resident the needed degree of security and familiarity. Then why aren't they recognized for that accomplishment?

As a direct caregiver, I learned very quickly that I rarely heard when I did something well, but always heard when I "screwed up". There are few "miracles" in what we do. Our wins in the eyes of those who do not know our job seem very small. In actual fact those small wins, given the complexity of these individuals are major accomplishments. It is essential that the accomplishments of staff be recognized and communicated frequently. The only way I can be motivated to continue what I am doing is when I know that what I have done was important and worthwhile. If recognition is lacking, so will the initiative to be creative and attempt something new. If the positive is not noticed, but the negative is always commented on, then a person will not take a risk. Why risk, when taking a risk means that the chances are high of creating many errors before reaching the desired goal and the errors seem to be what is always seen and commented on.

THE PRIMARY CARE MODEL

OVERVIEW

Primary care has become an effective model for long term care facilities. It allows a facility to achieve the goals of quality of life for the residents; to establish staff and team efficiency and effectiveness; to coordinate interdepartmental involvement in resident care; and to minimize bureaucracy leading to effective organizational problem solving.

The effect of primary care is to place the responsibility for resident care and problem solving at the team level. With the introduction of primary care, the long term care industry has found the needed vehicle to effectively meet its mandate. In the past staff/resident assignments were randomly made, with minimal consistent contact by any one staff with any one resident. The authority structure of most organizations placed limitations on the freedom of direct line staff to adjust and define the care routine. Communication between shifts and other departments was minimal and general. When an organization is divided into departments, not teams, problems and information must take a long and complicated path from the Nurse's Aide to the Registered Nurse in charge of the unit, to the Director of Nursing, to other department heads, to their staff, and back before being resolved.

Primary care in essence flattens the organization and divides a large facility into distinct smaller units. Each unit operates with autonomy, having its own full and part time staff. Consistent staffing to the unit does not just encompass the nursing department, but every other department that may have contact with the resident – recreation, adjuvant, social services, housekeeping, dietary, etc. This concept encompasses the full dynamics of team involvement. Consistent staffing at all levels not only enhances communication and problem solving, but ensures that everyone is aware of specific issues of individual residents, improving the quality of care provided. In essence, these units are self-contained, almost as small facilities within a large facility. They have control over budgetary expenditures, equipment, supplies, even personalizing the home's philosophy of care to fit the specific needs of the resident population living on that unit.

COMMON PRIMARY CARE TERMINOLOGY

Staffing Pairs   – this involves a full time staff member and that person's regular part time replacement.

Primary Teams   – the six staff (3 full time and their 3 part time replacements) who are assigned to one resident group.

Resident Grouping   – the number of residents assigned to the primary team is determined by dividing the number of full time equivalents on duty during the day shift into the number of residents on the unit.

Care Team   – all members of a unit, encompassing all departments – RN, RNA, nurse's aide, recreation, housekeeping, dietary, maintenance, etc.

OBJECTIVES OF PRIMARY CARE

The objectives of primary care are as follows:

- to decrease the number of staff working with individual residents in a 24 hour per day, seven day per week period.
- to provide each resident with a staff advocate on each shift.
- to maximize individualized/personalized resident care.
- to ensure consistency in care and programming.
- to provide a consistent link between the resident and all departments.
- to enhance team functioning and organizational problem solving.

TEAM CONFIGURATION AND STAFF ASSIGNMENT

An organization that randomly assigns direct line staff to resident care each shift, creates the possibility of twenty one different caregivers being assigned to one resident over a seven day period (a different nurse's aide each shift, each day). This inconsistent assignment of direct line staff to residents has been demonstrated to have the following effects:

- an increase in resident aggressive or withdrawn behaviour
- an increase in custodial care
- a loss of resident individuality
- a lack of consistency in care
- a creation of "islands" among departments and shifts
- wasted time and resources
- increased pressure on those who are conscientious about their work

When primary care is implemented those problems can be overcome. With this model there is the ability to reduce the number of staff caring for any one resident to six in a seven day period. Successful implementation of this model focuses on the staff's master rotation schedule.

A true master schedule does not only identify the consistent scheduling of full time staff, but also identifies:

a) a consistent scheduling for part time staff
b) the primary team this staff member belongs to
c) the unit this person is on
d) the group of residents the staff are assigned to

a) Part Time Schedule

We must first discuss the part time schedule. During each rotation (the number of weeks required to repeat the same schedule pattern), the master schedule always has the same number of replacement shifts that must be filled (excluding sick time and vacations). Consistent part time assignments can be accomplished by simply taking the number of replacement shifts and evenly dividing them by the number of part time staff available. Each part time person is then assigned the replacement shifts of one full time staff member throughout the rotation. In this way the master schedule creates paired groupings of staff: a full time and that person's consistent part time replacement. It is important now that staffing pairs be matched into primary teams.

b) The Primary Team

The primary team consists of six staff – three full time and their consistent part time replacements. All six are assigned to the same group of residents. To create a balanced primary team without assignment conflicts, it is important that a full time staff member working the day shift is matched with another full time staff member who is simultaneously working the evening shift, and another who is simultaneously working the night shift. In this way, when one primary worker (part or full time) is on the day shift, there will always be one on the evening and night shift. The result is to have one of the six primary workers on duty on each shift, every day of the week.

c) Resident Groupings

To create resident groupings, the resident population of a unit is simply divided by the number of full time equivalents on duty during the day shift. For example, if a unit consisted of thirty five residents and there are the equivalent of five staff on duty during the day shift, there would then be five groupings of seven residents, each called primary groups.

It is imperative that these groupings not be randomly chosen. The groupings must be arranged by the team based on the care requirements of individual residents. Each primary group should represent a mixture of heavy to lighter care, balancing the work load and the room location of each resident to prevent undue running. If a consistent complaint is made by a number of staff of one group, then that is an indication that the groups are unbalanced and there needs to be some adjusting to make them even.

Implementing primary care on a unit with thirty five residents and five full time staff equivalents on the day shift would create five primary teams, each comprised of six staff (three full time and three part time) and seven residents to each staff assignment.

It is important to stress with direct line staff that being assigned to a group of residents does not mean that they are solely responsible for the care of those residents. Care is still completed as a team, sharing responsibility for baths, beds, etc. Should a primary worker be off the unit to lunch or coffee and his/her resident requests to go to the bathroom or be served her lunch, the fact that the resident's primary worker is not present does not absolve other staff of taking on those duties. Care is the responsibility of the entire team on the unit. The role of the primary worker goes beyond just the physical care and standard responsibilities.

ROLE OF THE PRIMARY WORKER

The primary worker is responsible for the following:

1. To accurately know the resident under his/her care
This not only involves the day-to-day care issues but goes much further. The primary worker is responsible to uncover and communicate issues pertaining to the resident's personal history; emotional, psychological, physical, environmental, spiritual and social needs; current and past problems that may impact on the resident's present situation; physical, social and mental abilities; and personal idiosyncrasies that must be met to provide personalized/individualized care.

2. Assessment
The primary worker is a major contributor in the completion of any assessment – functional, recreation/social, psychological, medication, activities of daily living, etc.

3. Advocate
One of the most significant functions of the primary worker is acting as an advocate for specific residents. The primary worker supports, represents or speaks on behalf of the resident regarding any decisions concerning routines, living arrangements or needs, care conferences, moves, treatments, etc.

4. Evaluation
The primary worker is utilized as a major resource in evaluating the effectiveness of programming and care strategies implemented by the care team, as well as the overall response of the resident to living within the facility.

The primary worker assumes a role similar to that of a family member or significant other who is caring for an older person. In caring for an older client in the community, any professional (physician, physiotherapist, counselor, community health nurse, etc.) would rely heavily on the family caregiver as a source of information; a focal point in providing instructions so that they can be clarified for the older client at a later date; someone who will ensure that things are followed through and someone who will be required to observe and report the results of any treatment or programs initiated. Likewise, the primary worker provides the same resource and supports.

The primary worker becomes an ideal medium to define need, relate history, give instructions, follow–through on interventions, evaluate effectiveness, and detail problems. In essence, the primary worker becomes the resource to other professionals who have less contact with a specific resident, but who need detailed information in order to function effectively. Having a consistent primary worker on each shift ensures that this assistance and information is always available.

Diagrammatically, the primary worker's relationship to the resident and other departments can be represented as follows:

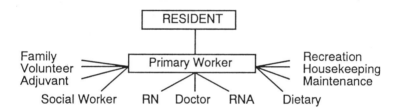

An immediate response by some professionals when looking at this diagram is that too much "authority" is given the nurse's aide. In actual fact the primary worker does not have authority, but becomes a resource person for other staff. If the doctor has placed a resident on a certain medication, it is logical that during his rounds, he would want to talk to the primary worker on duty to see if there has been any change in the resident's behaviour or functioning. Likewise, if maintenance is planning to change the faucets in a resident's washroom, it would make sense to inform the primary worker. If the resident cannot tolerate the added stimuli, it may be more practical to do the work at a time when the resident is not in the room, rather than to upset her. Should the recreation staff want to know the best time for a resident's activity, the primary worker becomes the most logical resource.

Imagine the support to volunteers and family that primary care provides. Volunteers are not only assigned specific residents, but can also be linked with that resident's primary worker, guaranteeing that there will always be someone there to support them while on the unit. Similarly, family will see the same staff members involved with their parent, providing significant support and contact for information.

An additional benefit of primary care involves evaluation and accountability. Under the primary care model, when direction or an intervention is discussed at a care conference, there is now a specific and limited number of staff required to follow through. For example, if it is decided that a resident is capable of learning to feed herself with a spoon using her right hand, then the primary workers involved with that resident are required to implement the intervention. It is obvious that the rapport of the primary worker with that resident would be a significant asset in motivating her to attempt this degree of independence. Secondly, there are now only 6 staff (the primary team) involved in giving instructions on what has to be done. This ensures more consistency in what is asked of the resident, by staff who have learned how to communicate with her and are sensitive to her physical and psychological limits. In this way demands placed on the resident are more realistic.

Under the primary care model, problems encountered or sudden changes in the resident's ability to perform need not wait until the next care conference. The primary team can immediately discuss the response of the resident with the registered staff or physiotherapist in order to adapt what is being asked. Even if the primary worker should be off the unit during certain meal times, she is responsible to have another staff member assist the resident to learn to use a spoon and is to ensure that the needed instructions are provided. Now the possibility for success of any program or intervention has greatly improved.

Under primary care, evaluation of what has been requested is more thorough and accurate. When registered staff are charting the resident's progression, they need only talk with the primary worker. At a care conference when the care plan is reviewed, the primary worker will be able to comment on how well the resident has responded.

Furthermore, primary care ensures accountability of resident care. When things are not followed through or completed properly, then specific staff can be identified and approached in order to clarify their role or determine problems in performing what is required. Under this model, staff become very aware that they are expected to take ownership for their actions and all realize that how they perform their job has a tremendous impact on the quality of care provided. Now individual staff who have difficulty with certain duties can be easily identified so that they can be assisted in improving their performance.

POTENTIAL CHALLENGES TO PRIMARY CARE

When a hoyer lift is introduced to a unit, staff are given a specific set of instructions on how to use it. It doesn't matter where that lift is used, in what facility, which unit, or who is using it, the instructions are universal. That is not the case with primary care. Even though guidelines for implementation can be provided, each unit will need to fine tune the concept to adapt it to the idiosyncrasies specific to that unit. Many of these issues will not surface until the model is introduced. It must be stressed to all staff and managers that "problems" are the only way to know how to adapt the concept. Then and only then can steps be taken by the team to decide what needs to be done. The following are some common issues encountered in the implementation of primary care.

a) Off Shifts

Evening and night shift usually change the configuration of the resident assignment. A unit that has a different number of staff on duty with each shift – i.e. five staff on the day shift, four on evenings and two on nights – will have to adjust the assignments for the off shifts. On the day shift, a thirty five bed unit will have a staff/resident assignment of seven residents (the basic number for each primary team), but on the evening shift when four staff are on duty, three staff will be assigned to nine residents and one will be assigned to eight residents. This is not as complicated as it appears. The number of staff on each unit is consistent each week, therefore once the assignments are made, they also become consistent.

The resident assignment on evening shift is not randomly chosen. It is based on the primary team. The four staff on afternoons must each be assigned the seven residents that would comprise their normal grouping as though they were working the day shift. That will leave one group of seven residents left (a thirty five bed unit would have five groupings of seven residents each). The remaining group of seven residents is then divided evenly among the four staff. Two residents from that group to three staff and one to the fourth. Once this resident grouping is created, it need not be changed. Staff know that each time that specific week is repeated in the master schedule, they will be assigned the same additional residents. (With a master schedule, once a pattern is identified it is repeated that week in every rotation.) In this way, staff would know their assignment well in advance and have an opportunity to familiarize themselves with those residents before moving onto the evening shift, ensuring consistency in care and programming.

The night shift is not as crucial and can easily be divided. If there are only two staff on duty and thirty five residents on the unit, each staff member would be assigned their normal resident grouping and consistently divide the remaining residents.

b) Sick Time and Staff Vacation

In the event of sick time and staff vacation, the most appropriate replacement strategy is to have a part time member of that primary team replace the person who is off. In this way the primary team stays intact. In a unionized facility where staff replacement is based on seniority, some complaints may arise. This can be overcome by negotiating that for the first nine months of the year, part time staff within a primary team would replace staff who are off sick or on vacation. If by the ninth month, there are discrepancies where lower seniority part time staff have more accumulated hours than those of higher seniority, then those of higher seniority are called to replace any staff for the last three months until the imbalance is rectified.

Replacement for long term disability is the easiest to accommodate. Those shifts can be assigned to any staff, as long as it is the same part time or group of part time each week for the duration of the person's illness. Consistency in staffing is therefore maintained.

It is consistency in staff replacement that is the priority in primary care. Given the realities of a 24 hour operation, staff must be aware that the master schedule cannot guarantee 100% consistency no matter what efforts are employed. There will always be a time when a staff member who is not part of a specific primary team or even a regular member on a unit who will be assigned a group of residents she does not know. Under primary care, the impact of that occurrence on care and team functioning will be minimal. Random assigning of staff becomes the exception rather than the rule. At least with the degree of consistency that can be maintained, there are enough regular members on the unit during that shift to provide the "new" staff member the necessary direction and support, ensuring that the routines and approaches are maintained.

c) Double Booking

With any master schedule there will be times when members of the six person primary team (those assigned to the same group of residents) may be working the same shift for one or two days every rotation (possibly when one staff has moved to the day shift and the other is about to switch to the evening shift). Even though this is a break in the scheduling pattern, it will be a consistent occurrence, repeating itself every five weeks (the length of the master schedule rotation). That staff member would then be assigned to the free group of seven residents. Even though not ideal, that staff member will know which residents will be under her care during that period, this person now becomes a member of a second primary team. Knowing that, allows this staff member the opportunity to prepare for the resident care to be given. Again it is the consistency that is important. Staff have advanced warning about who they will be caring for and know that specific assignment will be repeated in every rotation of the master schedule.

d) Utilizing Four Hour or Spot Shifts

Many units regularly schedule four hour shifts. Other facilities on certain shifts will have an extra staff member on duty (spot shifts), either to accommodate scheduling changes, or specific activities regularly arranged on that unit for that day of the week. The four hour and spot shift staff do not become direct members of the primary team. Instead, their role is to assist the primary workers. They would be assigned specific tasks – i.e. bathing certain residents. Their duties will vary depending on the needs of the team or certain residents.

For example, a staff member working the four hour shift may be asked to bath a resident the same day each week for three weeks. On the fourth week, that person may be required to bath a different resident in that time slot. The rationale for this change is dependent on the resident or primary team. During the first three weeks this resident's bath was straightforward and could be completed by anyone with only minimal direction provided by the primary worker. If during the fourth week it was decided at the care conference that this resident could be taught to assist in her bath, then the primary worker would want to be involved in that task rather than the four hour staff person. This again would ensure consistency in approach and effective evaluation of the success of this intervention.

e) Length of Primary Team Assignment

The length of time staff are assigned to one group of residents can vary from one to three months and depend on a number of factors. That decision is left to the discretion of the care team.

It is best when first initiating primary care to begin at the low end. Initially many staff may be unsure of what is expected of them. Even though the concept may be understood, its implementation and effect is not yet known. Much of the "old" way of thinking about resident care may result in some staff seeing this as "more work". They may resist the concept of primary care only because they believe that the length of time assigned to a resident group and the associated work load is unfair.

It is best to begin with a one month trial period. After that month the assignments can be reviewed and the decision made on what is an appropriate duration. If after that month there are a number of complaints about the work load by staff assigned a specific resident group, then it is not the time factor that is the issue, but the imbalance in the group arrangements. In that instance, the groups need to be re-adjusted until having one group of residents really doesn't matter. When staff begin to realize that the groupings are all about the same in the amount of time required, the number who need to be lifted, the number who are difficult and so on, the length of time assigned to a group becomes irrelevant.

Suggested Steps in Implementing Primary Care
1. Establish consistent part time scheduling.
2. Assign the same part time to the same full time each week.

3. Create the primary teams by matching staffing pairs who work opposite shifts (when one is on the day shift, the other is on the evening and the other on the night shift).
4. Create resident groupings by dividing the number of residents on the unit by the number of full time staff equivalents on the day shift, arranging the groupings by resident care and location on the unit.
5. Assign primary teams to specific resident groupings.
6. Consistently assign staff of other departments to the unit (housekeeping, recreation, dietary, etc.).

SUMMARY

We all have a limitation that frequently gets in the way of almost everything we do. That limitation is very simple – we are only human.

Although it sounds ludicrous to make such a statement, admitting to being "human" at times doesn't seem to be acceptable in our business. There is often an expectation that admitting to one's limitations is an admission of weakness.

I have always found the attempt to deny our human limitations very interesting. While teaching in a diploma nursing program, I began to think that some faculty had been out of the work force too long when they told the students, "You leave work at work and home at home". We have identified that the "best" staff we have are those with the greatest amount of caring and compassion. If you have that level of emotion invested, how do you shut it off at 3 o'clock?

Imagine the following:

You have had an unusually long, hard day at work/
You are exhausted/
You go home, to find you have to cook supper/
After supper,
You have to clean the table, dishes, the floor and the kitchen/
Nothing seems to be going right/

Your children are irritable and resisting going to bed

Everything you planned to do that evening is an hour
    behind/
You finally get the kids to bed and settled/
You have to work the next morning at 7 am
That means you have to be up by 5:30 am//
You are exhausted
You're asleep as soon as your head hits the pillow/

At 11:30 pm
Your youngest is awake
Vomiting his "socks up"/
He is vomiting until 3 am/
You get a few more hours sleep/

You go to work for 7 am/
You are assigned a number of mentally impaired residents/
You walk into your first resident's room
And find he is covered in feces/
You clean him up/
You walk into your second resident's room
She is nude and wants to leave the building/
Your third residents spits in your eye/

It is 7:45 in the morning/
How are you?

Fit to be tied. You express to your peers "These residents are driving me crazy." Some reply "they don't bother me".

On a day such as this, you need someone to say to you "Are your residents safe? No one is going to fall out of bed? Then get off this unit and take 15 minutes to have a cup of coffee and cool off."

In some facilities that freedom does not exist. There is a fear that when certain staff (those who are "negative") learn they can have an extra break on a bad day, they will have a bad day every day. This fear of a small number of staff abusing this freedom often results in no one receiving it.

That means that even if you are our "best staff", you are treated as though you are not, and are told to go back into that room without a break.

What is the result of such a restriction? I don't believe a good staff member would become abusive towards the resident just because she was sent back to the resident's room. What a positive staff member will do is possibly say or do things that she would normally not say or do. The question that arises is how long? How long can you have such situations occur where you are not supported and still maintain your enthusiasm?

You have heard the word "burnout". Burnout is not a disease. It is a reality of this job. It is only those who care that "burn out". If you don't care about your job, if you see it only as a job that provides an income, then you will not invest any time, energy or thought. You just "do".

If you are truly involved in your job, you become a high risk to "burnout" if the supports are not in place to encourage you to perform at your optimum. Any mentally impaired resident can exhaust any one staff member. That resident exhausted his family who had a lot more caring and compassion than any staff. How can a staff member be expected to function on her own without supports?

An effective team process is the key to quality care. The team (encompassing all levels of staff and management) must be supportive and provide staff the needed resources to allow them to function. It is important that staff be free to admit that certain residents will tax their patience, resulting in their losing their objectivity. There has to be the freedom and acceptance of one's limitations. At times, it is best when caring for the hard to handle resident that a staff member simply say to another "I have had enough for today, you go in and take care of her for awhile."

We have frequently established in this text that all that may be done for some of the repetitive behaviours of the mentally impaired is to make them tolerable. That may mean not changing the resident as much as the staff's reaction to the situation – determining how long one can deal with that person's behaviour, before passing that resident onto someone else, is an effective intervention in many situations.

Being human must be an acceptable quality of all staff. We don't work with these residents for only a few weeks. We work with them for the rest of their lives. That can be years of doing the same thing and dealing with the same behaviours. If the team and the facility cannot be supportive of its own people, then the desired level of care cannot be provided.

FAMILY

Many families have successfully cared for a mentally impaired mother or father for a considerable period of time before admitting them to our facility. The response by family to mother's illness and present needs depends on a number of factors;

1. The existing family dynamics.

How family members related prior to the crisis with mother will dictate how well they deal with mother now. If family members were tight-knit most of their lives, then dealing with the problems encountered with mother now will probably be positive. If family were always distant, then the situation where mother is in need may not be sufficient to draw them together, leaving only one or a few family members to deal with the entire situation.

2. The communication and problem solving ability of the family network.

If family members did not communicate effectively or were unable to solve any previous crisis well, they will not deal with this situation well. In such a situation, feelings are usually held in and not discussed until they become uncontrollable. When these feelings are expressed during emotional tension, things are said that are not meant, only distancing family members further. Likewise, if the problem solving ability of family members is not effective, then crisis intervention is all that remains. In crisis intervention the situation is not logically thought through, but dealt with only when there is no other choice. Such a process only results in taxing existing energy and resources, and a lot of time. These fits of harried intervention can easily lead to premature exhaustion on the part of certain family members.

3. The support systems available to the family caregiver.

If the person responsible for the brunt of the care and decision making does not have an effective support system in place, then exhaustion becomes a reality. The ability of the caregiver to take care of herself is mandatory in such a situation. If the family caregiver cannot admit and accept that she is only human, she will not provide for herself the necessary outlet to release much of the emotional tension experienced. The result is to lose patience with the situation encountered due to the physical, mental and emotional exhaustion experienced.

4. The degree and severity of the symptoms of the mentally impaired family member.

If mother's symptoms go beyond basic care (help with eating, dressing and toileting), but involve aggressive outbursts, wandering or safety hazards, then the ability of family to provide 24 hour supervision for an extended period of time will break down.

I have always admired how long families have dealt with some very trying circumstances in taking care of their mother or father before considering admission to a long term care facility. As staff in a long term care facility, we only see families when their ability to care for mother has been exhausted. We have not seen what the family has done for the past year or two or longer in attempting to keep mother in the community. If we only knew the whole story of such diligence, our understanding of the varied family response to the existing situation would be clearer.

Imagine:

A mentally impaired resident under your care/

Take that person home/
Where you alone are required to provide care/
Twenty four hours a day
Seven days a week
For three months/

Dealing with all meals/
Dressing and undressing each day
Concerned about wandering/
Incontinence
Safety/
Coping with repetitive behaviour by yourself/

Your normal routine
How you have always done things in the past
Has now been altered/
Your activities have been curtailed/

It is difficult to find anyone who is willing to sit with this
        resident while you are out
Friends don't seem to visit as much
They find it so hard to deal with this resident when they
        are over/

Each day, every day
The same behaviour/
The same care/
The same routine/
How will you be at the end of the three months/

By the time some families have reached our facility they are
exhausted. Family are not just overwhelmed by the daily care
issues – meals, laundry, toileting, etc. – but also with an intense
emotional tension as well.

Many families experience an emotional crisis created by a
situation that has seen mother deteriorate slowly over time. It is
the emotions encompassing the loss that creates the problem. If
the situation could only be dealt with on a logical basis it would
be so easy. Unfortunately, if logic were the way that family
reacted to this crisis, I would be concerned about the relationship
they had with their mother all of their lives, or that the emotions
they are experiencing are being buried only to surface at a later
date.

Emotions in this situation are to be expected and it is hard
not to let those emotions get in the way when solving the
problems encountered. It can always be said that emotions bar
logical thinking. When I work from my heart, my head seems to
be in neutral.

The scenario, above of you taking care of a mentally
impaired resident for three months in your own home, was taking
care of someone else's mother. It is easier to be objective when
dealing with someone else's family member. Make that person
your mother. Not many caregiver's I have met are able to do with
their mother what they do with their residents. The objectivity can
so easily be lost. In dealing with our family it becomes hard not to
let the emotions get in the way of our thinking.

FAMILY'S RESPONSE TO THE DISEASE

Living with a family member who is mentally impaired can be a time of constant family & grieving. Grieving each loss experienced. Often the death of that loved one after a long bout with the disease has attached to it little outward emotion. By the end, that emotion has usually been spent.

All of the stages of grief are experienced by family at some time.

1. Denial

A common response by some family is out and out denial, a belief that mother will get better. Some family seem to constantly talk and act as though what mother has will eventually go away – refusing to accept that the disease cannot be stopped and will only worsen with time. Families who continue to deny what is happening become the ones who will not accept mother's behaviour, believing that if she only would try harder she could do better. This family usually pressures mother and staff to achieve unrealistic goals. The inability of either to accomplish what the family expects results in increased friction between mother, family and the staff, making the situation only worse.

2. Blaming

Other family members may present a different response called blaming. In blaming, the family uses the environment mother is in (the facility) or the staff as the cause for mother's behaviour. Families interpret the day-to-day changes seen in mother as staff's inability to do the job needed. The transition period after admission is usually the time staff will see this response. It is difficult to accept that the decision to move mother was the main cause for her ability and behaviour to deteriorate. There is enough guilt in making that decision without considering the consequences of it. To compensate, the emotion is displaced onto staff – it is their fault that mother is worse, they are not doing a very good job.

Certain family members may direct that blaming on themselves as they see an improvement in mother the longer she is on the unit.

Mother is living with you
Each meal you constantly struggle for her to feed herself/

You invest considerable energy to keep her independent
That energy is strong the first few meals
What about the 117th meal in a row?
Finally you find it easier to do it for her/

Mother is admitted to the facility/
A short time after admission
You discover mother is feeding herself/
Something she would never do for you/

How would you feel?

It is easy to blame yourself for mother's deterioration. You do not realize that the reason for staff's success is that no one staff member works with your mother for more than a few meals. This sporadic contact allows staff a better opportunity to maintain their objectivity and persistence. Unfortunately, when emotions entangling your vision, it is easy to believe that if only you had tried harder, maybe mother would have been able to function at home like she is now. Such an admission only conjures up that possibly there are other areas where "you failed" in your attempt to take care of mother, meaning that it was your fault that she was admitted. You didn't do a good enough job. It is so easy to feel guilty.

3. Anger
     A further response to the situation encountered by family is anger. Anger can be directed at a number of sources. One is towards oneself for the feelings one is experiencing. Family can encounter two conflicting feelings at the same time – love and hate.

> "Mother I love you, but I hate what you have become and what you have done to our relationship."

At times this can create the wish – "If only mother were dead." Once that thought is encountered, family become angry at themselves for being so cruel and selfish.
     Anger can also be directed at staff. They become an easy target for the building emotions encountered. It is impossible to vent or even express your feelings to your mother now that she is

ill, so you vent those feelings on those most available – staff. The only neutral targets.

Family often express to me "I hope the staff understand." Under normal circumstances if family experience a problem they elicit the appropriate amount of emotion in relation to the severity of that problem. However, when emotionally tense and the same problem is encountered, the emotion expressed is exaggerated in comparison to the severity of the problem. Family will often state that when they "blew up" over a small thing, they didn't know what happened. Once the emotions start coming out, they felt as though they couldn't stop them. It was like a dam broke and it all flooded out. The response staff experience from family may not be related to what is happening at that time but is a culmination of feelings built up over time that just needs the right opportunity to be expressed.

4. Depression

The last feeling and probably the one most frequently encountered is depression – helplessness/hopelessness. Helpless that there is nothing family can do to change the situation for my mother and hopeless, there is nothing you as staff can do either. This feeling often leaves family in an awkward situation. Each time they visit, the more hopeless it seems. This makes visiting an unpleasant experience. Over time visits become less and less desirable and the frequency drops to avoid such bad feelings.

FAMILY & GUILT

The chronic feeling of family through this whole experience is guilt. The best definition of guilt is a belief that if only I were bigger, stronger, smarter, and faster I could have done it as planned. Like staff, family have difficulty admitting that it is okay to be human.

The problem families often encounter is that "their plan" does not go as scheduled. That "plan" is the family's expectations of what is going to happen, how it will be dealt with, who will do it, what it will take and for how long. It is this expectation of an orderly manner in which things are to go that often motivates the family to undertake some very trying situations. The problem with some families is that "the plan" may be rigid, with little or no thought of alternatives should that order be disrupted. Knowing the mentally impaired, there is no such order and a rigid plan will always fail.

Once the "plan" fails, time, resources and energy are exhausted and other decisions have to be made. The guilt surfaces when one of those alternatives are undertaken. "If only I could have been _____, I could have made it work." There is no decision family can make that has "good" feelings attached to it. Leave mother alone in her home when she is impaired and family are riddled with worry about her safety and physical state. Take mom into your home and the family becomes upset about the disruption in their own lives. Admit mom to a long term care facility and the family feels as though they have abandoned her. For family the only choice they have is which of the "bad" feelings they want to live with. It becomes the lesser of three evils.

KNOWING WHAT IS HAPPENING

In my counselling practice, there are two things that I do with families – grief counselling and teaching. It is amazing how many families do not understand what is happening. This lack of knowledge of the situation can have some devastating results:

1. Subjectifying the symptoms
Family may interpret mother's behaviour subjectively, believing she can control what she says and how she acts – "Mother can remember an event that happened 30 years ago, but she refuses to remember that I visited yesterday" or "Mother could remember my name yesterday. She is just trying to make me feel guilty." Without understanding the dynamics of the disease process, such a subjective response to mother's actions can only alienate family further.

2. Fear of one's own mother
Not knowing what to do or what may be triggering mother's behaviour, family may find each visit is more and more uncomfortable, as they become afraid of what mother may say or do. Some family member's have stated that mother is "cruel". Not learning how to deal with mother's outbursts may result in fewer and fewer visits.

3. Feelings of inadequacy

When mother was home, family did everything for her. Now that she is in the facility, there is nothing to do. If family are not given a role in mother's care, you may find that all they are left with is a simple visit. With nothing to do and with mother incapable of carrying on a coherent conversation for any length of time, visits may dwindle to only special occasions.

4. Overwhelmed

The disease and admitting mother to a long term care facility are both new experiences. Dealing not only with a changing mother, but also encountering a number of other older people who are severely disabled either physically, mentally or both, becomes a situation that many lay people cannot deal with.

WHAT TO DO

There are options available to help family deal with such situations:

1. Education and Support – Family need to learn about the disease and about the facility. Scheduling a regular Family Night is valuable, where families have an opportunity to meet once a month for an educational session. The Alzheimer's Society is probably the most active family group and very powerful in its ability to teach others about the disease and provide family member's with the needed supports.

2. Role – Family members need to be a part of mother's care while she is living in the facility. That requires staff to show the family the areas of care they can participate in, teaching family about the activities in which mother is involved, having the family participate in unit activities like Smorg night, special outings, picnics, family days, etc.

3. Resource – The people who may know the lady in our care best are the family members. They can provide the needed pieces of who this person was and how some of the behaviours we are seeing now may be related to events in her past. If the family has done the care, then they can provide direction of what is effective and what is not.

If the family is not invited into our facility and shown how they fit within the framework of things, we will lose them. Then staff will wonder how they are going to compensate for the family's absence.

SUMMARY

This is a people business. We care for people in crisis (our residents), we relate to people who are directly affected by our care (family) and we expect people to do a job that requires special skills and personal fortitude (staff). Emotions, needs, rewards and a purpose, all play a part in deciding the success of what is done. Our days of custodial care are over. We are challenged now to establish for all involved a quality of life. A stimulating challenge. a rewarding opportunity.

Chapter Fifteen

EPILOGUE

Some ask "How do you know that the world of the mentally impaired is as you described?" I don't! The challenge in this text has been to take a world of chaos and place it into logical terms. There is no way to be accurate in what is described. All that we can do is attempt to understand that person's world in whatever way possible. The closer we can come to the experience, the more effective our interventions and care will be.

This is not an exact science. Nothing we do in the health care field can be measured and dissected to clearly paint the whole picture of what each individual experiences when in such a crisis. Ours is a profession that is based on professional hunches. An attempt to pin down some direction. If it were easy there would be no challenge.

We have only begun to understand the mentally impaired. Their world is still a mystery, but the key to unlock that mystery is in view. The fear is that before we find a cure for Alzheimer disease, we will find a way to slow it down rather than stop it. That may be a blessing to those mentally impaired who are in level one, still able to function, losing only minimal cognitive functioning. Those in level two, in conflict with reality, living in two worlds at the same time, dependent on others and level three, those totally out of contact with reality and who can respond only to custodial care may not be so fortunate. The ability to medically slow the disease will raise some serious moral and ethical questions – do we take measures to have a person live 20 years with the disease by the treatment devised, or do we let the disease run its course, where the person will live only 11 years? There will be no easy answer, but a dilemma we will certainly face.

TO THE FUTURE

Long term care has gone through a major transition over the years. Initially long term care facilities had a resident population that averaged 74 years of age and included a clientele that required minimal supports. The picture began to change in the late 1980's when the resident population averaged 85 to 87 years in age and consisted of a clientele physically frail and incapacitated requiring supports in all areas – physical, psychological, emotional, behavioural, social and environmental. This changing clientele taxed the available resources of all long term care facilities – the physical structure of the building had to be changed to accommodate wheelchairs, walkers and physically frail individuals; staffing numbers needed to increase just to meet the physical needs of the resident population; staff expertise had to be enhanced to understand what was happening and what needed to be done; support services, physiotherapists, occupational therapists, social workers etc., had to be utilized to assist staff; the assessment and analytical process had to become more sophisticated, and so on. Some facilities have not dealt well with this transition. Some found themselves attempting to surmount so many difficulties with such a changing resident population that the effect was disastrous on staff morale and eventually care. We are reeling, but coming back, finally getting a hold on what is needed and finding a path to achieve it. However, we are in another transition.

This new transition involves the mentally impaired elderly. Most facilities today have a resident population that is evenly divided – 50% of the residents are cognitively well/physically disabled and 50% are mentally impaired. The demands are changing rapidly for facilities to develop the skills and resources needed to handle the increasing population of mentally impaired residents. The problem of caring effectively for the mentally impaired elderly will not be one that lessens, but only intensifies.

Most long term care facilities are finding that their waiting lists are bulging with clients experiencing some degree of mental impairment and fewer and fewer applicants require only physical supports. Within time most facilities will find that 75% of their resident population will be mentally impaired, with some facilities specializing in this clientele only.

The physically frail older person is not as quick to go into a long term care facility today as he was in the past. Now there are an increasing number of community services available that encourage an older person to remain at home. Meals on wheels, transportation systems, friendly visiting, chronic home care, nursing visits, day hospitals, retirement centres and so on, have all been proven effective and well–utilized. The list is impressive and still growing. Within a short time we will find considerable commonalty between communities in terms of what is offered. All of these alternatives make moving into a long term care facility an option that is needed only when all others have been exhausted. A person will find he needs to enter a long term care facility only when he requires more care than can be found within the community, or when his financial status does not allow him to maintain his independence at home. This is happening already.

Those who will need long term care are the mentally impaired elderly – level two, the high risk for wandering behaviour, aggressive outbursts, repetitive behaviour, etc., the ones difficult to care for in a family member's home even with community support services available. This person needs care and supervision 24 hours a day, where the greatest safety problem may be at night. The safest and most appropriate location for a majority of level two mentally impaired will be in a long term care facility.

This is a "catch 22" situation. As the population of mentally impaired residents in long term care facilities increase, the cognitively well will be less willing to move in.

We will see further specialization in our field – becoming the "experts" in caring for the mentally impaired elderly. Either we prepare for our role now in a conscious effort to develop our resources and staff for this clientele, or we prepare for it when we are struck full force with the need.

There are some exciting things happening and some very skilled and creative individuals making them occur. No matter what you do, you are probably breaking new ground. No matter what you do, you are a pioneer in determining the best direction to care for the mentally impaired.

There will be struggles and battles that must be won to tap further resources. There will be a need to change many philosophies on the approach to be taken with this clientele. Ardently, you can be the main force in that change. I hope that this book has provided you with some guidance and direction in your quest to develop the best quality of life for this very special population. Beyond the specific suggestions, I have attempted to challenge you to be creative, to take chances in seeking new avenues towards better care. Go Ahead. Accept the challenge – your initiative is needed and will make a difference.

Addendum

24 HOUR PROFILE

The intention of the following team assessment is to provide a profile of a specific resident's functioning level over a 24 hour period. The purpose of the information is to:

1. Identify changes in functioning noticed between shifts (days, nights and evenings)
2. Identify the resident's strengths and weaknesses
3. Identify successful techniques or approaches employed by certain staff in each area

Instructions:

Step 1 - This questionnaire is to be initiated by a staff member who best knows the resident to be assessed. That staff member is required to complete the Supportive Data section for the shift that most contact is made with this resident. Be as specific as possible recording any supportive data you believe appropriate to describe this individual's functioning in each area. Write as though the person who is reading it knows nothing about the resident being discussed.

In the space under Supportive Data include the following:
- pattern of behaviour (time of day, equipment to be set in a specific manner, specific items used, etc.)?
- when you have seen changes (will or will not function)?
- what do you say or do to the resident to assist the person to function?
- have you found any effective means to encourage the person to function?
- how can you tell if the individual is being pressured and it is best not to perform the task at that time, or to assist the person in completing the task?

Step 2 - The complete form is then reviewed by each shift (days, afternoons and nights) during a care conference adding to the information provided.

Step 3 - Once completed, a list of care issues is extracted and the guidelines outlined in the Supportive Data becomes the basis for the care plan.

24 Hour Profile

Resident's Being Assessed _____   Date of Initial Assessment _____
Initial Assessment Completed By _____   Date Reviewed By Day Shift _____
                                                               Evening Shift _____
                                                               Night Shift _____

	Day Shift	Supportive Data	Evening/Night Shift

ACTIVITIES OF DAILY LIVING   Yes No
1) MEALTIME
   - needs assistance (explain)   ( ) ( )
   - easily distracted (how is this dealt with)   ( ) ( )
   - can only handle few items at a time   ( ) ( )
     (which & in what order)
   - any special arrangement or items?   ( ) ( )

2) HYGIENE   Yes No
   a) BATHING
   - co-operative in tub (if no explain)   ( ) ( )
   - needs assistance (explain)   ( ) ( )
   - any special arrangements or items?   ( ) ( )

Evening/Night Shift

Supportive Data

Day Shift

b) TEETH/HAIR

	Yes	No
- needs assistance (explain)	( )	( )
- requires articles to be handed to him/her	( )	( )
- requires articles displayed only	( )	( )
- Cooperative during procedure (if no explain)	( )	( )
- any special arrangements or items?	( )	( )

c) DRESSING

	Yes	No
- requires assistance dressing or undressing (explain)	( )	( )
- requires articles displayed	( )	( )
- requires articles to be handed to him/her	( )	( )
- problems with specific articles of clothing	( )	( )
- can pick own clothing from closet	( )	( )
- any special arrangements or items?	( )	( )

Supportive Data

Evening/Night Shift

Day Shift

d) TOILETING

	Yes	No
- specific times (which?)	( )	( )
- needs to be checked (when?)	( )	( )
- how does he/she communicate the need to go to the washroom		
(tell you or by what actions?)	( )	( )
- any special arrangements or items?	( )	( )

AMBULATION

	Yes	No
- gait unsteady (describe gait)	( )	( )
- needs to be checked, will exhaust self	( )	( )
(what time of day and what is done if unsteady?)		
- wanders (identify time and specific area)	( )	( )
- how do you deal with the wandering?		

Supportive Data

Day Shift

COMPREHENSION

Yes No

- understands instructions (if no explain) ( ) ( )
- responds to his/her name (first, last or
  nickname?) ( ) ( )
- can identify staff or family members
  (who and how often?) ( ) ( )
- can identify all objects
  (if no, what and when?) ( ) ( )
- find way around unit - room, washroom,
  dining room, lounge ( ) ( )
- what must you do to help this person
  understand what you are saying or what
  you want done?

BEHAVIOUR

Yes No

In each area where (yes) is checked describe
what the resident does and how you deal
with it

- restless ( ) ( )
- repetitive behaviour ( ) ( )
- destructive ( ) ( )
- disturbing behaviour (to who?) ( ) ( )
- hoarding (what, from where?) ( ) ( )
- verbally/physically threatening others ( ) ( )

Supportive Data

Day Shift   Evening/Night Shift

SOCIAL SKILLS   Yes No
- can relate to others (will talk to who,   ( ) ( )
    when and about what?)   ( ) ( )
- will help others (who & when)   ( ) ( )
- relates well to new people   ( ) ( )
    (if no, explain what happens)   ( ) ( )
- participates in group activities?   ( ) ( )
    (what and when)

ACTIVITIES   Yes No
- will perform specific chores on the unit   ( ) ( )
    (what and when?)
- be involved in specific games, hobbies   ( ) ( )
    (what, when and for how long?)   ( ) ( )
- will read or look through books/magazines   ( ) ( )
- enjoys music, t.v. (what and when?)   ( ) ( )

BIBLIOGRAPHY

Birren, James E. and Schaie, K. Warner; Handbook of The Psychology of Aging, Second Edition, 1985, by Van Nostrand Reinhold Company Inc.

Burnside, Irene Mortenson; Nursing and The Aged, 1976 by McGraw–Hill Inc.

Butler, Robert N. and Lewis, Myrna I.; Positive psychosocial approaches, Aging and Mental Health, the C. V. Mosby Company, 1977, and revised edition 1983.

Cohon, Gene D.; The Brain in Human Aging, 1988 by the Springer Publishing Co.

Cone, John D. and Hawkins, Robert P.; New directions in Clinical Psychology, Behavioral Assessment, 1977, by Brunner/Mazel Inc.

Epstein, Charlotte; Learning to Care for the Aged, 1977 by Reston Publishing Company Inc.

Fabiano, Len; Birminham, Joesphine, et al; Ontario Association of Homes for The Aged; Guide to Caring for the Mentally Impaired Elderly, 1985 by Methuen Publications.

Fabiano, Len; Working With The Frail Elderly; Beyond The Physical Disability, 1985 by ECS Publications.

Fabiano, Len; The Nurse Manager (& Others Too) in Long Term Care; 1988 by ECS Publications.

Fabiano, Len; Mother I'm Doing The Best I Can, Families of Aging Parents During Times of Loss and Change; 1989 by ECS Publications

Gray, Barbara and Isaacs, Bernard; Care of The Elderly Mentally Infirm, 1979 by Tavistock Publications.

Gwyther, Lisa P.; <u>Care of Alzheimer's Patients</u>, A Manual for Nursing Home Staff, 1985 by American Health Care Association and Alzheimer's Disease and Related Disorders Association.

Health and Welfare Canada; <u>Alzheimer's Disease</u>, A Family Information Handbook, 1984 by Ministry of Supply and Services Canada.

Heston, Leonard L. and White, June A.; <u>Dementia</u>, A Practical Guide to Alzheimer's Disease and Related Illnesses, 1983 by W. H. Freeman and Company.

Hogstel, Mildred O.; <u>Nursing Care of the Older Adult</u>, In the hospital, Nursing Home and Community, 1981 by A. Wiley Medical Publication, John Wiley & Sons.

Mace, Nancy L., and Rabins, Peter V.; <u>The 36-Hour Day</u>, A Family Guide to Caring for Persons with Alzheimer's Disease, Related Dementing Illnesses and Memory Loss in Later Life, 1981 by The John Hopkins University Press.

Powell, Lenore S. and Courtice, Katie; <u>Alzheimer's Disease</u>, A Guide for Families, 1961 by Addison-Wesley Publishing Company.

Reisberg, Barry; for families, <u>A Guide to Alzheimer's Disease</u>, for spouses and friends, 1981 by The Free Press, New York.

Roach, Marion; <u>Another Name for Madness</u>, The Dramatic Story of a Family's Struggle with Alzheimer's Disease, 1985 by Houghton Mifflin Company.

Rodman, Morton J. and Smith, Dorothy W.; <u>Pharmacology and Drug Therapy in Nursing</u>, Second Edition, 1979, 1968 by J. B. Lippincott Company.

Ross, Marvin; The Silent Epidemic, A Comprehensive Guide to Alzheimer's Disease, 1987 by Hounslow Press.

Springer, Sally P. and Deutsch, Georg; Left Brain, Right Brain, 1985 by W. H. Freeman and Company.

Wedding, Danny and Horton, Arthur MacNeill, Jr. and Webster, Jeffrey; The Neuropsychology Handbook, Behavioral and Clinical Perspectives, 1986 by Springer Publishing Company Inc.

Whitehead, J. M.; Psychiatric Disorders in Old Age, A Handbook for the Clinical Team, 1974 by Harvey Miller & Medcalf Ltd.

Williams, J. Mark G.; The Psychological Treatment of Depression, A Guide to the Theory and Practice of Cognitive-Behaviour Therapy, 1984 by The Free Press, New York.

Wolanin, Mary Opal, and Phillips, Linda Ree Frallich; Confusion, Prevention and Care, 1981 by The C. V. Mosby Company.

Yurick, Ann Gera and Robb, Susanne S. and Spier, Barbara Elliott and Ebert, Nancy J.; The Aged Person and the Nursing Process, 1980 by Appleton-Century-Crofts.

Zarit, Steven H. and Orr, Nancy K. and Zarit, Judy M.; The Hidden Victims of Alzheimer's Disease, Families under Stress, 1985 by New York University Press.

Index